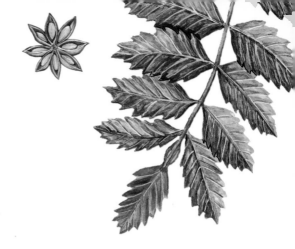

GROW
YOUR OWN
SPICES

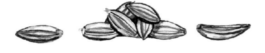

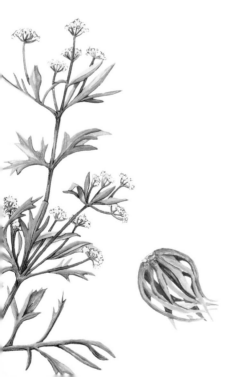

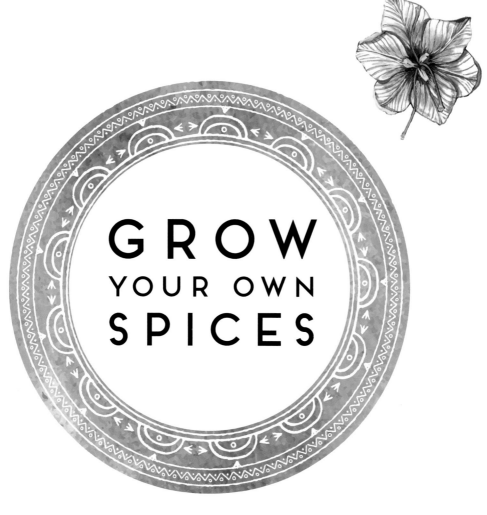

GROW
YOUR OWN
SPICES

HARVEST HOMEGROWN
GINGER, TURMERIC, SAFFRON, WASABI,
VANILLA, CARDAMOM,
AND OTHER INCREDIBLE SPICES
NO MATTER WHERE YOU LIVE!

Tasha Greer

with **Medicinal Usage Tips**
from Lindsey Feldpausch, RH

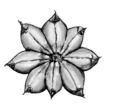

COOL
SPRINGS
PRESS

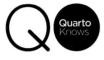

Brimming with creative inspiration, how-to projects, and useful information to enrich your everyday life, Quarto Knows is a favorite destination for those pursuing their interests and passions. Visit our site and dig deeper with our books into your area of interest: Quarto Creates, Quarto Cooks, Quarto Homes, Quarto Lives, Quarto Drives, Quarto Explores, Quarto Gifts, or Quarto Kids.

Inspiring | Educating | Creating | Entertaining

First Published in 2021 by Cool Springs Press, an imprint of The Quarto Group, 100 Cummings Center, Suite 265-D, Beverly, MA 01915, USA.
T (978) 282-9590 F (978) 283-2742 QuartoKnows.com

Cool Springs Press titles are also available at discount for retail, wholesale, promotional, and bulk purchase. For details, contact the Special Sales Manager by email at specialsales@quarto.com or by mail at The Quarto Group, Attn: Special Sales Manager, 100 Cummings Center, Suite 265-D, Beverly, MA 01915, USA.

25 24 23 22 21   1 2 3 4 5

ISBN: 978-0-7603-6802-2

Digital edition published in 2021

Library of Congress Cataloging-in-Publication Data

Names: Greer, Tasha, author.
Title: Grow your own spices : harvest homegrown ginger, turmeric, saffron, wasabi, vanilla, cardamom, and other incredible spices -- no matter where you live / Tasha Greer.
Description: Beverly, MA, USA : Cool Springs Press, 2021. | Includes index. | Summary: "Grow Your Own Spices shows gardeners of all skill levels how to grow their own spices, including ginger, turmeric, saffron, cumin, and many more"-- Provided by publisher.
Identifiers: LCCN 2020032353 (print) | LCCN 2020032354 (ebook) | ISBN 9780760368022 (trade paperback) | ISBN 9780760368039 (ebook)
Subjects: LCSH: Spice plants. | Spices. | Gardening.
Classification: LCC SB305 .G68 2021 (print) | LCC SB305 (ebook) | DDC 633.8/3--dc23
LC record available at https://lccn.loc.gov/2020032353
LC ebook record available at https://lccn.loc.gov/2020032354

Page Layout: *tabula rasa* graphic design
Illustration: Greta Moore
Photography: Tasha Greer, except Shutterstock on page 6 (center), 19, 20, 42 (top and bottom), 53 (top), 72 (top), 75, 93, 103, 111, and 123.

Printed in China

The information in this book is for educational purposes only. It is not intended to replace the advice of a physician or medical practitioner. Please see your health-care provider before beginning any new health program.

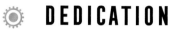 # DEDICATION

For the Sharweed family: Because you shared your beautiful culture, homegrown food, and friendship so freely during my formative years, I was able to write this book.

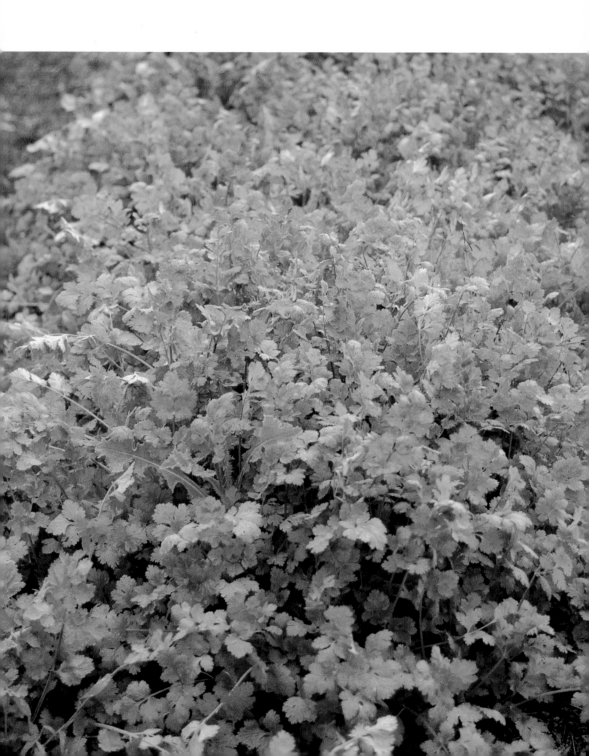

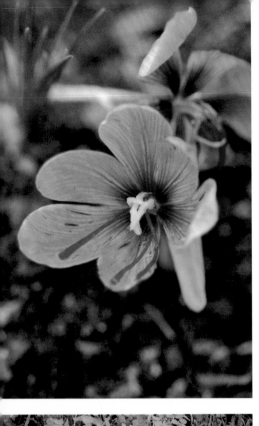

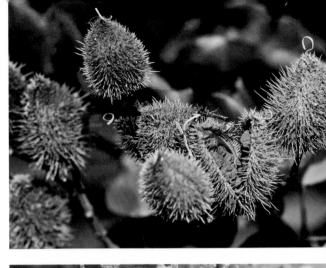

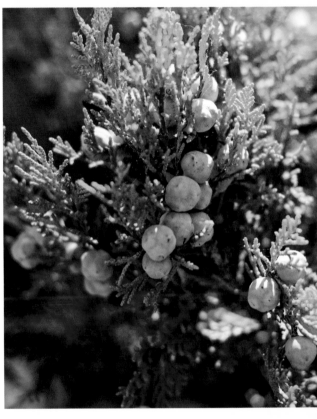

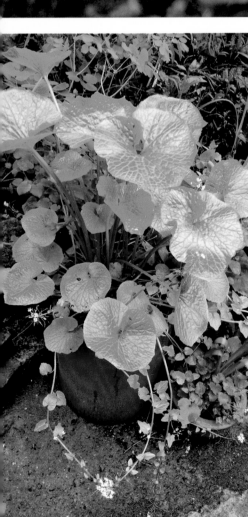

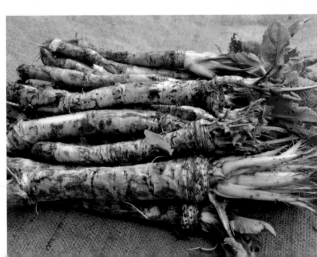

CONTENTS

INTRODUCTION

SPICE: THE FINAL FRONTIER IN MODERN HOME FOOD PRODUCTION

There's been a huge resurgence in the number of people growing food at home. Square Foot gardens, container herb gardens, backyard orchards, rooftop farms, community gardens, and chicken coops are taking over the landscapes of our modern lives. Simultaneously, more people are using herbs and spices to proactively support health.

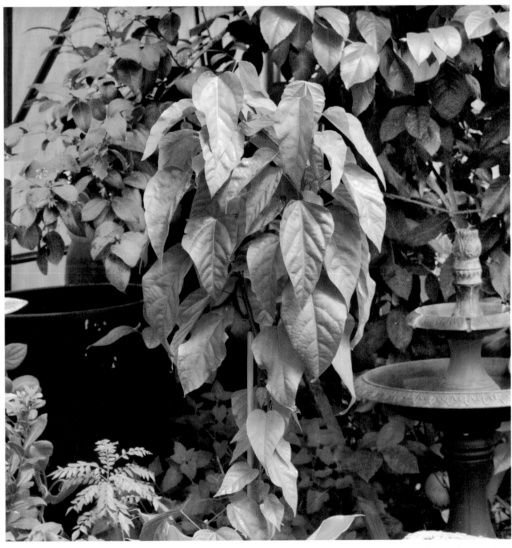

While the techniques required to grow many spices, including this annatto tree, were once a spice trade secret, this once-coveted knowledge is now available to home gardeners.

In some ways, this homegrown food and health movement is like stepping back in time. We're returning to our organic roots, making compost, planting heirloom seeds, eating foods fresh and in season. We make teas and tinctures to manage stress, aid digestion, and support our well-being. We flavor and color food naturally, as our ancestors did.

Yet, this movement is also distinctly modern. We grow vertically, on rooftops, in basements, in hot houses, and with electricity. We use scientific precision in plant propagation, fertilizing, soil care, and disease and pest prevention.

SPICE GROWING SECRETS

Despite our advances, there's one area of home food growing that novice and skilled gardeners still leave mostly to commercial producers. Of course, I mean the subject of this book, growing spices. Spices are like the final frontier in home food production.

Don't get me wrong; gardeners do dabble on the edges of spice gardening now. We grow ginger in pots, let dill go to seed, start garlic in fall, and more. However, even when we grow most of our own vegetables and herbs, we still tend to purchase the bulk of our spices in dried, processed forms.

There's a good reason for this. For ages, spice trading was so profitable that growers zealously guarded the secrets of plant propagation and spice care. In fact, there are many historical accounts of intrigue, espionage, murder, and wars over the spice trade.

Thankfully, those historical protectionist attitudes have changed too. Today, growing spices has become part of our public domain—no longer relegated to the role of intellectual property or trade secrets. Spice plants and seeds are available from suppliers around the world. The knowledge of how to grow spices is widely dispersed for free in blogs and videos.

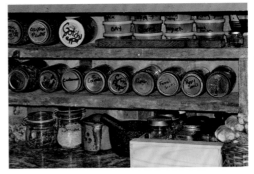

My personal homegrown spice collection is stored in sealed jars and containers for year-round use.

As we know, not every bit of information on the internet can be trusted. Also, environmental conditions have a big effect on spice plant health, so not all the information is applicable to every climate.

This book is meant to help distill that abundance of information into simple, practical methods that will work for most gardeners. It also aggregates that information for over thirty spices in one place.

PRESERVING OUR GLOBAL CULTURAL HERITAGE

For the record, I'm a gardener, food lover, and someone who cares about my health and our planet. I assembled this spice gardening collection, for all of you with similar loves, as a simple place to start. I also recruited my friend, herbal medicine expert, Lindsey Feldpausch, RH, to offer medicinal tips to help you cultivate better health too. However, this book is only possible because cultures and communities around the world have cultivated these plants, and the knowledge to grow and use them, for thousands of years.

As such, this work is meant as an homage to the incredible natural and human history embodied in the aromas, tastes, and health benefits of these durable delights. It is my

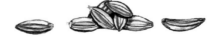

hope that the information in these pages will help you grow spices at home. My deeper wish, though, is that by growing your own spices, you'll feel a sense of gratitude, as I do, for the cultural and natural diversity responsible for this spice collection.

Unfortunately, it's impossible to appreciate that diversity without also being aware that it is threatened not only by climate change, but by a climate of cultural inequality. Spices, in my experience, are a kind of window to the world. They can serve as a regular reminder and celebration of our rich global heritage and our need to preserve it.

Growing spices alone will not change the world. Growing our awareness and capacity to care for cultures different from our own absolutely can. As a gardener, I know that every plant I grow also grows me. Spices seem to have an uncanny ability to deepen my connection to the earth and all its inhabitants. I very much want this same experience for you.

FURTHER STUDY

In the same way that our homegrown vegetable movement blends our agricultural and cultural past and our technological present, this next phase of spice growing will be too. If you want to journey deeper into the histories, cultures, and uses of the spices described in this book, I invite you to visit my website www. simplestead.com.

There you'll find links to the wonderful resources I've come across in my research, plus recipes and other tasty tidbits, to help foster a deeper connection to the spices you grow and use. If you have "spicy" experiences, please leave comments so all of us spice lovers can learn from you.

DEGREES OF DIFFICULTY

Before we delve into the details of spice growing, let's cover a few administrative matters.

First, the organization of this book is loosely based on the difficulty of level of care. Truthfully, all these spices are easy to grow in the right conditions. The more "difficult" spices may require special treatment outside their native habitat. For example, some perennial spices need tropical or subtropical environments and may take a few years to fruit. That means you must care for them longer and create suitable microclimates for plant health.

Today, in cold weather, many of us use heat and humidifiers in our homes. In doing so, we create perfect overwintering environments for heat- and humidity-loving perennials. Sometimes, simply by taking advantage of our comfortable living spaces, we can grow exotic spices year-round.

Please don't let special requirements for care deter you. No sunny window? Try an energy efficient daylight-rated light fixture. Forgetful about watering? Set up a self-watering irrigation system. Too busy to fertilize? Use slow-release, organic fertilizer stakes. Even the most finicky spices can be made simple to grow with thoughtful planning and the right tools.

GENERAL GARDENING TECHNIQUES

Next, individual profiles will detail specific growing requirements. They'll also include suggestions to help each spice thrive just as it does in its native habitat. Besides those specifics, I'll aggregate information on basic gardening techniques at the start of each section to reduce your total reading time.

NEW AND SEASONED GARDENERS

Finally, this book is intended for use by new and well-seasoned gardeners. The organization of the sections loosely corresponds to the progression of skills needed to successfully grow the various spices. We'll start with relatively fast-growing spices raised from and for their seeds. Then we'll move on to plants

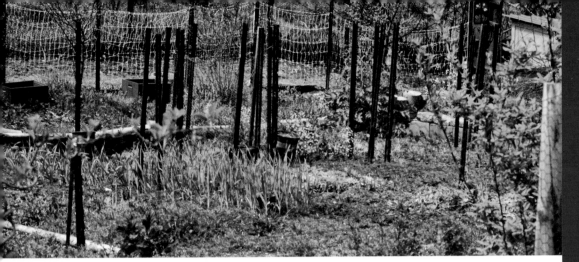

My own garden in the spring is filled not only with fruits and vegetables, but also herbs and spices.

grown for their underground parts. Finally, we'll end with perennial plants that require long-term commitment.

Within each section, the spices are further separated into subsections based on temperature or care requirements. For example, in the seed section, there is a subsection of spices that require cool conditions and another for plants that require warmer weather.

Beginners will benefit from using the book in sequence to build gardening skills while growing spices. Also, consider starting with the spices in each section that most closely align with your climate before you move on to the complexities of creating microclimates.

If you are an experienced gardener, you may want to focus on the spices that will challenge you to create the ideal conditions for optimal plant growth. Or take on multiple spices from each section simultaneously to put your skills to the test.

THE PERENNIAL QUESTION

With administrative matters attended to, let's quickly tackle a question that has boggled the minds of cooks, gardeners, and food lovers for ages.

What's the difference between herbs and spices?

Many people class herbs and spices together for good reason. They are both aromatic, have medicinal and culinary uses, and are consumed in small quantities due to their potency. Yet from a gardening perspective, spices are very different from herbs.

Herbs are the leafy green parts of plants that can be harvested at any point during their growing season for fresh use. They can also be easily dried to use later.

Spices, by contrast, require harvesting at specific points of plant development. Spices need specialized care such as ensuring cross-pollination or vernalization. Additionally, spices have unique processing requirements to preserve them for later use.

Don't be intimidated by these special requirements, though. We'll cover them in detail in this book. Plus, once you master growing spices, you'll have the skills you need to grow just about anything, including herbs.

Without further ado, let's start spice gardening!

BASIC SPICE PLANT CARE

Following are the basic care guidelines that will apply to most spices in this book. For any spices that deviate from these guidelines, alternate care instructions will be detailed in the individual spice profile.

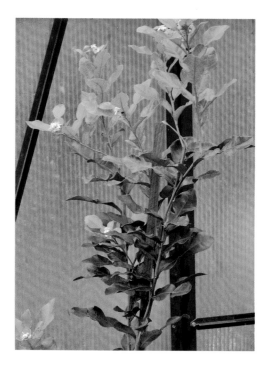

SOIL

Except for vanilla (which is derived from an orchid that grows in tree litter) every spice in this book grows well in quality garden soil or potting mix with good drainage. You can buy soil mixes or make your own.

My soil mix is equal parts native clay soil (sifted), aged compost, and leaf mold. The Square Foot Gardening mix (equal parts compost, peat moss, and vermiculite), commercially sold organic potting soil, or raised bed mixes also work well.

SOIL PH

The soil pH scale runs from 0–14, with 7 being neutral. A numeric reading below 7 is acidic and above 7 is alkaline. To effectively draw nutrients from the soil, plants require specific pH ranges (included in each spice profile).

Determine soil pH by using a pH test kit. If needed, opt for slow-acting soil pH amendments (pelleted, not powdered forms) to limit harm to soil life. Incorporate compost when you adjust pH to act as a buffer for plant health until the pH stabilizes. Or purchase soil mixes designed with the right pH to use in pots or raised beds.

SANITATION

Spices are susceptible to bacterial, viral, and fungal infections. Good sanitation minimizes risks related to these pathogens.

- Start with clean pots. Wash with soap and water.
- Then, soak in a bleach solution of 9 parts water to 1 part bleach for 10 minutes to sterilize.
- Dip garden tools in bleach solution for 1 minute between plants.
- Burn, or bag and dispose of, diseased plant matter to limit disease transmission.

RIGHT: If your fingers can't move through soil, roots can't either. Good soil is dark colored and easy to work by hand.

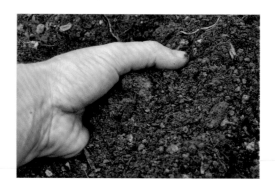

PLANT PESTS AND PATHOGENS

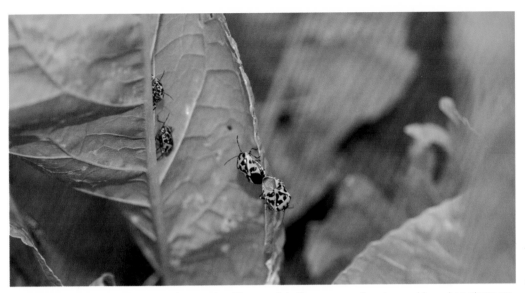

Harlequin bugs are a common pest of mustard and horseradish. They are usually only a problem when plants are grown in hot weather and plants are suffering from heat stress or drought.

Plants may be damaged or destroyed by herbivores (e.g., deer or rabbits), insects (e.g., leaf or root eaters), and pathogens (e.g., diseases). Risks vary by where you live and how you garden. You'll likely want to talk to other gardeners, or agricultural offices, in your area to get advice on specific risks and prevention planning. However, here are some broad areas to ask about.

Animals

Plants need protection from underground root-eaters such as voles, aboveground leaf-eaters like rabbits, aerial seedeaters like birds, and general destroyers like digging dogs. The use of fences, greenhouses, raised beds, protected container gardening, row covers, netting, or indoor gardening may help depending on your risks.

Insects

Healthy plants can repel insect attacks and better tolerate damage. Stressed plants are more at risk for insect infestations. Address minor pests by knocking them into a bowl of water, using insecticidal soap, or covering plants with netting or row covers. Reserve the use of insecticides—organic or otherwise—for extreme problems such as when multiple plants are simultaneously infested.

Pathogens

Fungal, bacterial, or viral pathogens cause plant disease. They spread through soil, garden tools, wind, insect dispersal, or plants and seeds. Prevention is key. Treatments may not exist or have limited efficacy.

Prevention practices such as buying disease-free seeds or plants, crop rotation every 1 to 2 years, and using high-quality soil amendments help. Maintaining diversity of soil life with regular applications of compost, mulch, and avoiding salt-based fertilizers and chemical toxins mitigate risks too.

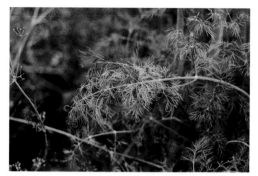

Discolored leaves indicate plant stress caused by lack of nutrients, inappropriate temperatures, water shortages, and insufficient light. The rainbow display on this dill plant indicates a shortage of water, warmth, and fertilizer.

Pale leaf color, yellowing of lower or inner leaves, too large or too small leaves, and leggy plants can all be signs of lack of light. Too much direct sun can cause pale and yellowing leaves leading to brownish or whitish scorch spots.

If you only need light and not heat, consider energy-efficient LED bulbs designed for growing plants. Fluorescent bulbs are less efficient. But they produce heat that can be helpful when growing tropical plants in cold climates.

LIGHT

Plants are designed to grow in natural sunlight. Even if you grow in containers or your plants need part shade, your results will be better if you grow outdoors whenever your climate will allow.

Indirect sunlight through windows or green-houses is filtered and may not be sufficient for year-round photosynthesis. Rotate (turn to the sun) window-raised plants to keep them from becoming lopsided. Supplement sunlight shortages using electric daylight-rated bulb fixtures.

FERTILIZER

Most of the spices profiled in this book require regular fertilizing. Fertilizer should be food-safe and organic when possible. Consider using one of the following options:

• Compost tea
• Liquid fertilizer
• Slow-release fertilizer stakes
• Pelleted granules

Avoid salt-based fertilizers as spices can be sensitive to salt accumulations. Also, amend soil annually with several inches of compost to maintain fertility and drainage capacity.

HOMEMADE COMPOST TEA

To make compost tea, soak 2 pounds (0.9 kg) of compost in a 5-gallon (19 L) bucket of water for 3–7 days. For smaller batches, use 1 ounce (28 g) of compost to 20 ounces (0.6 L) of water.

Use vermicompost (worm castings) if possible because it offers ideal beneficial bacteria for plant development. However, any compost aged a minimum of 6 months to minimize risks of pathogens will work. If the age of the compost is unknown, store for 6 months before use.

Apply 1 part tea to 9 parts water weekly, or as needed, for plant health. During peak growing times, if more fertilizer is needed, reduce to 1 part tea to 4 parts water.

MULCH

Mulch preserves soil moisture and adds nutrients as it decomposes. It's useful for most spices. However, keep these guidelines in mind:

- Don't apply mulch directly on trunks or stems to limit fungal and pest problems.
- For in-ground plants, apply 2 to 3 inches (5 to 7.5 cm) of mulch over an area several times larger than the mature plant's root zone will be. No mulch volcanoes!
- For potted plants, choose pots with room for sufficient soil and 1 inch (2.5 cm) of mulch.
- Cedar mulch may repel some pollinators. So skip it for plants that require pollination.
- Never incorporate mulch into the soil or it may rob plants of nutrients.

WATERING

Soil should be kept uniformly moist, but never waterlogged. Water slowly and deeply to encourage deeper root growth. Water a broad area around plants to retain moisture longer. Irrigation (e.g., drip or soaker hoses), olla pots, hand-watering, or misting systems are options to consider.

Newly planted seeds, transplants, and seedlings need daily watering of the top 2 inches (5 cm) of soil for the first several weeks until roots establish. Then water deeply whenever the top 1 inch (2.5 cm) of soil feels dry.

PLANT SPACING

Proper plant spacing is important for root growth and air circulation. However, if planting areas are sited for good airflow and have deep, fertile soil, you can use closer spacing for beauty and impact. More water and fertilizer might be required. Also, thin plants that show stress from crowding, such as yellowing or stunting, to prevent disease or pest infestations.

CONTAINERS

When appropriate, profiles will include suggested container or pot sizes. Spices are naturally adapted to grow in the ground and

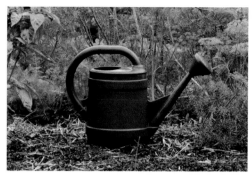

A large-capacity water can is a perfect tool for watering a small spice garden.

don't require a snug pot fit. However, larger-than-necessary pots require more soil, fertilizer, and watering. Also, starting plants in smaller pots may slow growth. That can be helpful to keep indoor-grown trees smaller for a longer period.

Potting soil mixes, rather than garden soil mixes, are preferred for use in pots as they are designed for better drainage. Unglazed terracotta pots are better for plants that need soil to dry between waterings. Plastic or glazed pots with drainage holes are fine for moisture-loving spices.

Periodically check on root development and be prepared to "pot up" before roots run out of room.

TEMPERATURE GUIDELINES

Each spice profile includes optimal temperature ranges for ideal growth. Also, the upper and lower temperature limits that spices can tolerate without risk of damage or death are listed.

Use the optimal temperature range for young plants and offer extra weather protection as needed. As healthy plants mature, they can tolerate temperatures that come closer to the upper and lower limits.

POLLINATION

Many spices come from the seeds or fruits plants. Sesame, for example, is the seed from inside the fruit of the sesame plant. Coriander seed is actually the fruit of the coriander plant. Mace is an aril, or membrane, located inside the fruit but outside the nutmeg seed.

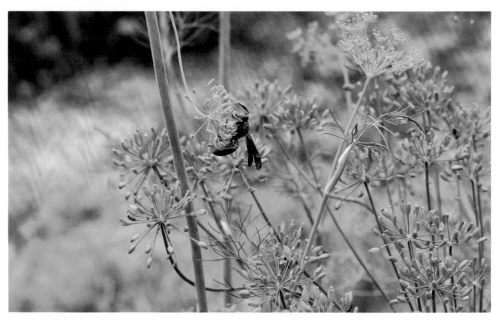

Pollinators such as wasps, bees, flies, butterflies, and more are needed to increase seed production even in self-fertile plants.

That's some fun spice trivia. But, what's important to understand is that fruit only happens when flowers are pollinated. Plant pollination needs its own book. For brevity, though, following is a short description.

- Male parts of a flower, called *anthers*, produce pollen that is used to pollinate female parts of a flower.
- The female pollen receptors, called *stigmas*, collect the pollen to send down the style to the plant's ovary.
- In the ovary, an egglike *ovule* is fertilized by the pollen.
- The fertilized ovule grows up to be a seed inside the fruit.

Types of Pollination

Some plants pollinate themselves without needing a second plant to reproduce. These self-pollinators come in two types.

1. *Completely Self-Fertile* plants have flowers that contain male and female parts and require no outside assistance to produce fruit.
2. *Pollinator-Dependent, Self-Fertile* plants have both the male and female flowers or parts necessary for self-pollination. Yet the pollen must be transferred from flower to flower by an outside party (e.g., insects).

Many plants can only produce fruit when they receive pollen from a second plant. These are called cross-pollinating. They also come in two types.

3. *Unisex, Self-Incompatible* plants have male and female flowers. Yet they also have features to prevent self-pollination and can only be pollinated by a second, similar plant.
4. *Sexed* plants have only male or female flowers and require a male plant be used to pollinate female plants.

Cross-Pollination Recommended

Even some *completely* self-fertile plants aren't perfect at self-pollinating. Pollination parts can malfunction, or the male and female parts can develop out of sync. Except for a few select spices, cross-pollination is recommended even for self-fertile plants. Locate several of the same kind of plant close together for cross-pollination.

Pollination and Spice Profiles

To ensure maximum pollination and fruit production, you'll need:

• an abundant insect population to transfer pollen from male to female flowers (e.g., by growing outdoors), or
• hand-pollination to ensure fruit production (when growing indoors).

Hand-Pollination

To pollinate by hand, rub a soft-bristled paintbrush over the male anthers. Then use that same brush to apply the pollen by rubbing the stigmas. One male flower can pollinate 3–5 female flowers.

Flowers open mainly in the morning, which is the best time to hand pollinate. Pollinate daily while new blooms are emerging. For cross-pollinating plants, collect pollen from one plant to apply to a different plant.

More Male Flowers

Many plants put out more male flowers than female. Male flowers may begin earlier and continue after female flower production ends.

Saving to Plant

To save seeds for planting, you also must prevent cross-pollination from plants that might alter the flavor of your spice plant. For completely self-fertile plants, isolation by at least 10 feet (3 m) is needed. For all others, aim for 300-plus feet (91-plus m) of separation.

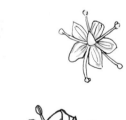
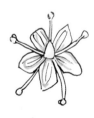

SECTION 1
FAST-GROWING SEED SPICES

Seeds are the foundation upon which agriculture was built. If our ancient hunter-gatherer ancestors hadn't realized that seeds could be cultivated for food production and storage, early farming communities would never have existed. Seed cultivation allowed humans to shift their energy from foraging activities to technological innovation. So growing spices from seeds is the perfect place to begin our journey.

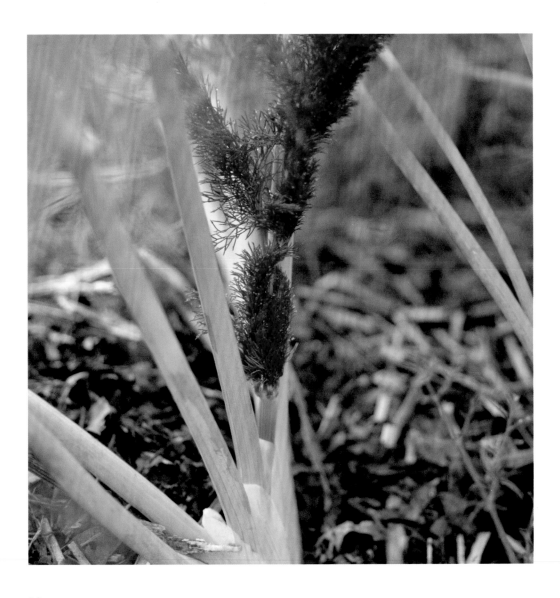

Even now, seeds are the foundation of our global diets. Intensive breeding, hybridization, and genetic modification have made most seed-based foods such as wheat, corn, and soybeans unrecognizable from the ancient varieties that fueled civilization.

Seed spices also played a prominent role in the origins of agriculture. For generations, growers have selected spice seeds for size, productivity, climate tolerance, disease resistance, and more. However, because the cultivation of these spices has remained mostly manual, the fundamental flavors and aromas of our spices are still similar to what our ancient human predecessors enjoyed.

Coriander, for example, has been used as a culinary condiment for over eight millennia. Yet the pungent, citrusy, earthy flavor we savor today is much like what pre-pottery Neolithic people used to add interest to their meals.

Poppy, dill, and cumin also made frequent appearances in ancient diets and agricultural cultivation. Fenugreek was an early legume that doubled as a spice. Sesame was among the earliest oil crops. In fact, every spice in this section has ancient roots.

Despite their early origins, seed spices are similar to technological masterpieces. They're like tiny hard drives that contain the genetic coding to build a new plant from scratch. Seeds are also living artifacts of the evolutionary history of thousands of years of collaboration between humans and nature.

Plus, a single spice seed, grown in good conditions, can become a stunning flowering plant that makes hundreds more seeds. Those seeds, when properly planted and cared for, can make tens of thousands of new seeds and plants. Talk about excellent productivity!

The truly incredible thing about nature, though, is that seeds are not just about reproduction.

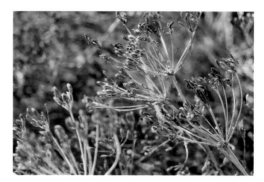

Seed spices, such as this cumin, are generally the easiest spices to grow.

Seeds are about sharing. Seeds simultaneously embody plant potential and are the perfect storage units for preserving flavor and nutrition for future eating.

When you plant a spice seed, you hold the ancient past and your culinary future in your hands. Don't be deceived by their small size or how easy they are to grow. Seeds are one of the most important technologies of all time, and we would not be here without them.

TECHNIQUES FOR STARTING SPICE PLANTS FROM SEED

Planting a seed is the *most* basic gardening skill. Yet it is also an art form. You can hurry up and get it done, or you can make it a mindful meditation and act of hopefulness.

Many of the spices in this section have *irregular germination* because they still retain their wild natures even after thousands of years of cultivation. For example, not every seed will germinate at the same time. Also, some seeds will grow in less-than-ideal temperatures while others will only start growing if conditions are perfect. These are part of nature's protection mechanisms to ensure survival of these plant species. For me, they serve as a reminder of our dependence on nature's intelligence and order.

With all due respect to nature, we still want a good harvest. Luckily, it's possible to encourage cooperation even when working with seeds that have minds of their own.

DON'T PLANT SPICES FROM YOUR KITCHEN

Seeds for planting are harvested from healthy plants with ideal genetics for reproduction. Spices for cooking were grown for production and harvested indiscriminately. As such, planting seeds from your spice rack is not the best way to grow spices at home.

SEED SELECTION

Seed savers harvest seeds from the plants that perform best in their specific environmental conditions. You'll have the easiest time growing spice seeds collected in your region or in climates similar to yours (especially related to humidity and weather fluctuations).

PLANT EXTRA

Due to the irregular and slow germination rates of many spices, you'll get best results if you plant extra seeds. Outdoors, plant 5–10 seeds in each hole. Indoors, use 3–5 seeds per pot or cell. Select your strongest seedlings to let grow. Use scissors to cut out all but the best seedling at the soil level.

SEASONAL PLANTING

Annual seed spices grow best in spring and early summer. Unless you have very moderate winters, fall planting is not ideal due to decreasing daylight hours, cooler temperatures, and a reduction of pollinator populations.

In areas with very mild winters, if spring is too hot or rainy, fall planting may be your only option for growing cool-season annuals. Fall-grown spices take a few weeks longer to harvest.

For biennial or perennial spices, late-summer planting is ideal as long as plant root systems have time to mature before cold weather sets in.

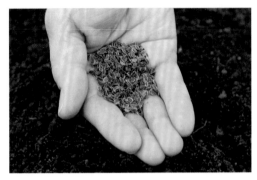

Annual seed spices, including dill, can be planted directly into the garden or started from seed indoors.

FIRST AND LAST FROST DATES

Apart from perennial fennel, caraway, and nigella, the plants in this section are frost sensitive. Plant outdoors after your area's last risk of frost and when optimal temperatures are achieved. Also, allow plenty of time for plants to mature to harvest before your area's first frost arrives.

GROW OUTDOORS

You *can* grow seed spices indoors. However, indoor yields are typically low, plants don't always set seeds, and pollination issues are common. Start plants indoors, then move them outside when the weather is right as a compromise.

BOLTING

Bolting describes a plant that is flowering sooner than it naturally should. Plants that have bolted produce fewer seeds. They may also be less aromatic and less medicinally potent.

Bolting is caused by excessive heat or dryness. To prevent bolting, use temporary shade cloth when temperatures soar and water more frequently with cool water. Mulch with light-colored materials to lower soil temperatures and retain moisture.

COMMITMENT TO CARE

A key difference between growing spices versus herbs is the time to harvest. Coriander

HARDENING OFF

Seeds started indoors require hardening off prior to planting them outdoors. Try one of these methods.

- Gradually increase the amount of direct sunlight plants get over a 7- to 10-day period. Start with 3–4 hours of morning sun and work up to a full day of light. Keep plants in partial shade with ideal temperatures otherwise.

- Transplant seedlings outdoors during a series of mild, cloudy days. Cover plants with floating row covers until they acclimate.

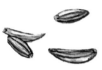

raised for its leaves takes four weeks to harvest. However, coriander raised for spice takes nearly four months.

Longer growing times mean prolonged risks for pests, pathogens, and inclement weather conditions to interfere with production. Continue to monitor plant health, and periodically water, fertilize, and hand-pick pests to keep plants healthy until harvest for best yields.

HOW TO PLANT A SEED

Gardeners tend to develop personal seed rituals and methods based on preference and experience. The following practices work for me and can be a good starting place for new gardeners. Or continue to use your favorite seed-starting methods.

1. Consider seed-planting instructions.
Every plant lineage, which is carried through its seeds, has nuanced variations in care requirements. The people who saved the seeds can often tell you exactly what conditions are needed to grow healthy plants. Read the descriptions and planting instructions on packets of new seeds carefully to glean important growing information.

2. Plant in soil mix.
I start seeds in the same soil mix in which I'll grow the plants. For potted plants, bagged

organic potting mix is my medium of choice. For outdoor transplants, I borrow soil from my garden.

3. Moisten planting medium.
Thoroughly moisten your planting medium before you add seeds.

4. Plant the seeds.
Plant the seeds at the depth indicated on your seed packet or in its spice profile in this book. For deeper-planted seeds, poke a hole with a stick to the right depth. Drop in the seeds and cover with soil. For shallowly planted seeds, place on top of soil, and then cover with a light layer of compost.

5. Maintain moisture.
After planting, keep the soil consistently moist. Don't let a crust form on top of the soil or it may prevent germination.

Water seeds and young plants like a gentle rain. Use a watering can or hose with a rosette head and a slow flow rate. Most seedlings initially put up two seed-breaking embryonic leaves called *cotyledons*. Next, the plant will begin to put on "true leaves" that look like small versions of mature leaves. When plants have several sets of true leaves, apply water to the soil, not to the plant's leaves.

6. Provide protection.

Maintain optimal temperatures. Protect young plants from weather extremes. For in-ground plants, cover with floating row covers, cloches, or cold frames. For potted plants, relocate them to a climate-controlled location during inclement weather.

TRANSPLANTING

All the plants in this section will transplant well if they have been grown in individual cells or soil blocks so their roots are not disturbed when transferring them to a new location. Avoid using the "pricking out method," which involves pulling roots from the starter soil. Transplant carefully before roots outgrow starter soil.

DIRECT PLANTING

All spices in this section can be direct planted in garden beds if the growing conditions are ideal. However, for warm-season crops in cool regions, or cool-season crops in warm regions, getting a head start indoors is preferable to direct planting.

WHEN TO HARVEST

Each profile includes pointers on when to harvest. However, your environmental conditions may affect your actual harvest time. Wet or windy conditions often necessitate harvesting immature seeds to avoid molding or seed loss. Or you may need to harvest early so birds don't steal your crop.

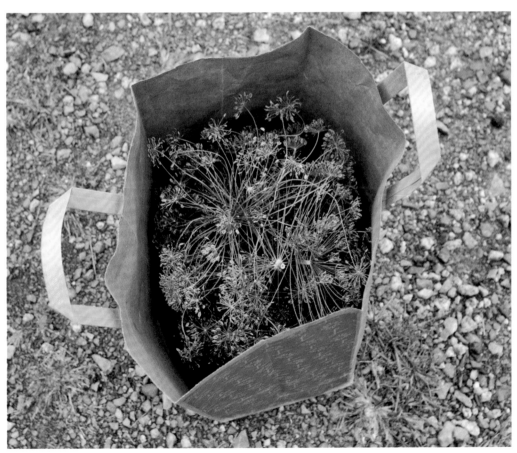

Seedheads can be stacked loosely in a paper bag to allow for good airflow. Don't compact the seedheads or bunch them together as that makes drying difficult. Leave the bag open while the seedheads are drying, if possible. Harvest on dry, sunny days and never directly after a rain.

REMOVING CHAFF

It's tedious to try to make your home-processed seeds as clean as commercially processed counterparts. Still, there are simple ways to get rid of most of the chaff in just a few minutes.

- Put your seeds into a large bowl or bag. Shake gently until most of the seeds settle on the bottom and larger chaff sits on top. Pick out the large chaff and discard.
- Then, when a breeze is blowing, step outside and gently drop your spice seeds from a high container to a low container. Lighter chaff will float away in the breeze while heavy seeds will fall into the container below.
- To remove dust, pour the seeds into a fine sieve. Shake lightly so dust falls through while the seeds stay inside.

GENERAL HARVESTING

To harvest, cut off the seedheads or seedpods and dry them inside a paper bag or on screened herb drying racks. To expedite drying, use an electric dehydrator on a low setting of around 90–100°F (32–38°C). Hotter temperatures may alter flavors and aromas.

For large harvests, use what I call the "candy wrapper" method for drying. Lay out a piece of air permeable fabric on dry ground. Place the seedheads or seedpods in the center. Roll the fabric and tie the ends like a candy wrapper. Hang the fabric roll, end to end, in a protected location with good air circulation until dry.

When the seedheads are dry, seeds may fall off. Shake these to the bottom or corner of your drying screen, bag, or candy roll. Then pour them into a container. Some seeds may remain on the head; pick off by hand or thresh to detach.

Some seeds in pods will crack or open when they're dry. Others may require that you use your hands to open the pods to free the seeds. For paprika, use the entire dried pod.

THRESHING

Seeds that don't easily separate from their plant parts require threshing. To do this for small quantities, put the harvested parts in a pillowcase. Gather up the opening and use that as a handle to beat the pillowcase on hard ground. Or tie up the opening, lay the pillowcase on a hard surface, and use a bat or stick to beat the pillowcase.

STORING SEED SPICES

Spice seeds, when stored in airtight containers and out of direct light, can last for three years or longer. Newly harvested spices will smell stronger after they rest in an airtight container for a few weeks.

For peak quality, package your spices in 3- to 6-month increments. That way you aren't exposing three years' worth of spice to the air when you need a small quantity for cooking or medicine.

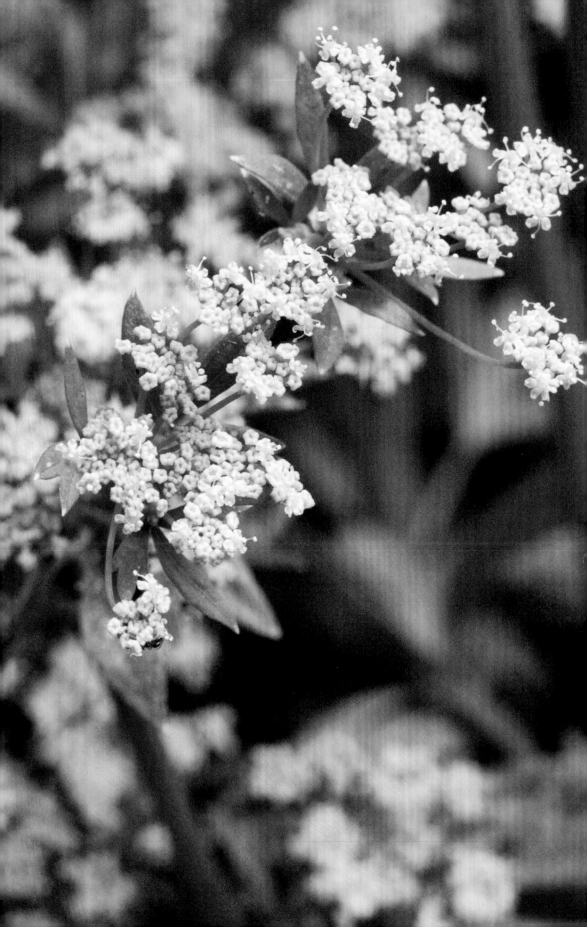

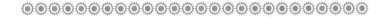

COOL-SEASON SEED SPICES

The seed spices in this section grow best when started and grown in cool weather. They require some additional protection and care during periods of extended heat to ensure good seed production.

CORIANDER	26
DILL AND FENNEL	28
FENUGREEK	30
MUSTARD	32
CELERY AND CARAWAY	34

< Biennial celery is a stunning specimen when it's flowering and seeding.

CORIANDER— THE ANCIENT SPICE THAT WENT VIRAL

CORIANDER IS ONE of the most ancient foraged and cultivated annual spices. Wild coriander was used by pre-pottery Neolithic communities over eight millennia ago as evidenced by seeds excavated in Israel. Seeds were also found in late Neolithic sites in Syria, Bulgaria, and Romania. In Egypt, 3,000+ year-old cultivated coriander seeds were found in Tutankhamun's tomb.

What's really incredible about coriander is that even without the Internet, it went viral early in human civilization. It spread from its native range across oceans and deserts to become a staple seasoning in every continent on earth.

Today, coriander is commercially grown in nearly every country with India, Russia, Mexico, Iran, and China being the top producers. Coriander grown in greenhouses has even been harvested by scientists in Antarctica.

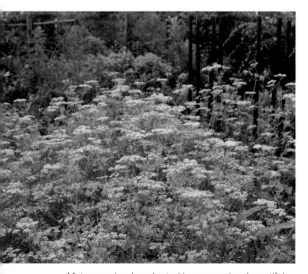

Mature coriander, planted in groups, is a beautiful choice for a flower or vegetable garden.

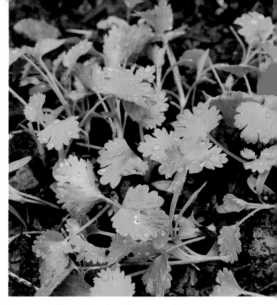

Grow seedlings close together to reduce weed pressure. As plants mature, thin the weaker plants to eat for their greens and roots.

CORIANDER CARE

Coriander is a compact plant with a taproot that grows low until flowering. It can produce three times more seeds if planted in close groups of multiple plants for cross-pollination.

Sow seeds ¼ inch (6 mm) deep. Plant outdoors when soil temperatures are consistently above 50°F (10°C). Plant extra and thin for leafy greens. Ideal final plant spacing as plants begin to flower is 3 inches (7.5 cm) apart on 8-inch (20 cm) rows for easy weeding. Or space plants 4 inches (10 cm) apart in all directions to suppress weeds.

At flowering, the central stem elongates and can reach several feet tall. Loosely tie several plants together for support in windy conditions.

European coriander needs minimal nitrogen. Argentinian or Indian coriander requires more nitrogen. Check with your seed provider for fertilization recommendations.

As a baseline of care, add 3–4 inches (7.5–10 cm) of compost and some aged poultry manure or worm castings to soil. Otherwise, fertilize and water regularly. Soil depth should be 8 inches (20 cm) for good seed production. In-ground planting is best, but coriander can be grown in 8-inch-deep (20 cm) pots too.

Excessive heat, inconsistent watering, and high humidity increase fungal risks. After flowering, plants are fairly drought tolerant.

Coriander flowers attract many beneficial insects.

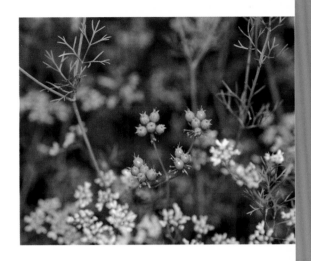

HARVESTING

In wet or windy areas, harvest seedheads when the pods have a reddish hue to avoid mold and shattering. Each plant can produce a tablespoon (15 ml) or more of seeds.

MEDICINAL TIP

Coriander's pungent flavor and citrusy scent come from its volatile oil content composed mainly of a monoterpene molecule, linalool. Research shows linalool to have strong anti-inflammatory and pain-relieving properties. Historically, coriander has been used as a sedative and to reduce anxiety.[1] Coriander's aromatic oils are also an effective carminative against stomach bloating and gas. As an antispasmodic, coriander can relieve cramping throughout the digestive system.[2] Add extra coriander seeds to all your gas-inducing dishes to mitigate their effects.

SPICE PROFILE

- **Names:** Coriander, Cilantro, Chinese Parsley
- **Latin:** *Coriandrum sativum*
- **Native to:** Southern Europe, Mediterranean, Western Asia; Landraces exist worldwide
- **Edible parts:** Leaves, seeds, and roots
- **Culinary use:** Pungent, earthy, citrusy flavor used in curries, meat dishes, sausages, soups, pickling, pastry, and liquor

GROWING CONDITIONS

- Cool-season crop; optimal seed starting 55–75°F (13–24°C); mature plant tolerance 20–85°F (-7–29°C)
- Provide afternoon shade and extra water above 80°F (27°C)
- Full sun; deep, fertile, well-draining soil; pH 6.5–7.5
- 4–14 days to germination; 30–40 days to leaf harvest; 100–120 days to seed harvest
- Partially self-fertile, cross-pollination recommended

ABOVE: *Each round coriander fruit contains two seeds. Use the entire dried fruit as the spice.*

DILL AND FENNEL— A TALE OF TWO SPICES

Dill is an annual plant. Fennel can be annual, biennial, or perennial depending on the variety grown. Both are similar in appearance and growing requirements with a few key differences.

Dill and fennel were cultivated by early Greeks and Romans for use in cooking, beverage-making, and rituals. These spices have also been used for millennia for culinary and medicinal purposes in China, Egypt, India, and the Middle East. Despite their worldwide reach, consumption today is most heavily concentrated in Europe.

Historically, these spices were believed to ward off evil or confer positive financial benefits on users. In modern times, we use fennel to ward off bad breath and dill to make our pickles "kosher."

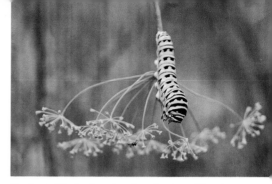

Swallowtail butterfly caterpillars feast on dill and fennel leaves and flower heads. Grow a few extra plants to promote a thriving butterfly pollinator population.

Commercial kosher-style pickles are now synonymous with dill seeds. However, the original barrel-made kosher pickles popularized by Jewish producers included kosher salt and vinegar. Dill seed was optional.

DILL AND FENNEL CARE

Technically, dill is completely self-fertile, while fennel is pollinator-dependent, self-fertile. Some seed-saving guides will say this makes fennel at risk for being pollinated by dill, but not the other way around. Personally, I've had fennel cross-pollinate my dill. The results were not tasty. As a precaution, I plant these two far apart, and at different times, to avoid muddling their flavors (both fresh for the next year and seeds for spice).

Sow seeds ⅛ inch (3 mm) deep. Similar to coriander, these can be grown in pots at least 8 inches (20 cm) deep but they will grow better in the ground.

Another controversy is whether dill and fennel require light or heavy fertilizer applications. In mineral rich soils (e.g., clay) amended with 3–4 inches (7.5–10 cm) of compost, fertilizer is not normally needed. Without compost or in sandy soils, add vegetable garden fertilizer or compost tea regularly.

In deep fertile soil, space plants 3 inches (7.5 cm) apart on 6-inch (15 cm) rows or on 4-inch (10 cm) centers. In shallow soil, allow one square foot (0.9 square meter) per plant.

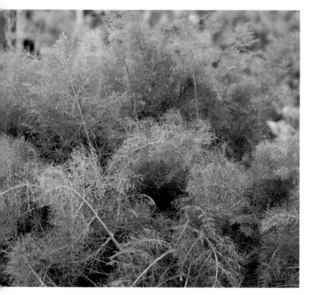

Lacy, fernlike bronze fennel makes a beautiful addition as a spice hedge or garden pathways. Plant densely for greater impact.

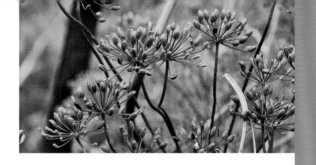

Both spices are hosts for swallowtail butterflies that eat the leaves. Grow a few extra plants as wildlife habitat.

Grow dill in your vegetable garden. It can tolerate a light frost but will be killed by freezing. Choose varieties labeled as "bouquet" or "seed" for peak production.

Fennel is best grown in a fennel patch. Annual and biennial fennel can produce tasty seeds. However, perennial wild or bronze fennel is the easiest to grow. Mature perennial fennel overwinters down to -10°F (-23°C). It reaches peak production in its third year and then declines. Start perennial fennel in late summer and harvest seeds the following summer.

HARVESTING
To limit seed loss, harvest seedheads when they show a slight brown hue. Dry in bags. Healthy plants can produce 1–3 tablespoons (15–45 ml) of seeds.

SPICE PROFILE
- **Names:** Dill, Dill Seed
- **Latin:** *Anethum graveolens*
- **Native to:** southern Russia and Mediterranean regions
- **Edible parts:** Leaves, seeds
- **Culinary use:** Slightly tangy, mild anise flavor used in pickling, sauces, and dressings

SPICE PROFILE
- **Names:** Fennel, Fennel Seed
- **Latin:** *Foeniculum vulgare*
- **Native to:** southern Europe and Mediterranean regions
- **Edible parts:** Leaves, stalks, seeds
- **Culinary use:** Strong anise flavor used in lamb and fish, sausage, soups, pickling, pastry, and making liquors

GROWING CONDITIONS
- Cool-season crop; optimal seed starting 50–75°F (13–24°C); mature tolerance 40–90°F (4–32°C) for dill, -10–90°F (-23–32°C) for fennel
- Protect dill from frost; protect young plants from heat
- Full sun to part shade; deep, fertile, well-draining soil; pH 5.5–7.5
- 7–14 days to germination; 20–40 days to leaf harvest; 100–150 days to seed harvest
- Self-fertile, pollinator-dependent, cross-pollination recommended

ABOVE: Dill seed is technically dill fruit. The dried seed is surrounded by a papery husk.

MEDICINAL TIP

Fennel is used as an expectorant and carminative. It can help break up mucous congestion in the respiratory system, aid the cough reflex, and act as a bronchial dilator to aid breathing.[3] As an aromatic bitter, fennel's activity on the gastrointestinal system reduces gas pains and spasms by stimulating digestion and relaxing smooth muscles. Fennel's gentle digestive attributes are used to relieve colic and indigestion in children. Traditionally, it is used as a galactagogue to stimulate breastmilk production.[4] Chew on fennel seeds or make a cup of tea to receive this plant's medicine.

FENUGREEK—PERFECT FOR PANCAKES

Fenugreek makes me think of childhood breakfasts. Back then, I didn't realize those aromatic seeds were responsible for the imitation maple aroma in American pancake syrup. These days, I don't eat much syrup, but I do grow fenugreek for its fragrance and culinary utility. I also use it as a tool to add nitrogen to the soil.

Humans have used wild fenugreek for at least six millennia. Its name means "Greek hay" and points to its early uses as fodder for livestock.

Today, fenugreek is renowned worldwide for its use in Indian cooking. It also plays a significant role in Ethiopian culture where it is used for livestock fodder, soil improvement, medicine, and as a key ingredient in berbere, a spice mix used to flavor popular dishes such as Doro and Masir Wot. Incidentally, those dishes are served with injera, a savory and healthy Ethiopian pancake.

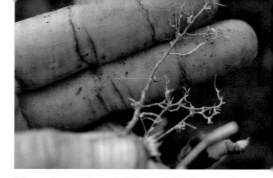

When a legume inoculant is used with fenugreek, rhizobia bacteria draw nitrogen from air in soil and attach it to plant roots. If the roots are left in the ground after harvesting, those tiny, white, spherical nitrogen nodules will decompose and feed other plants.

Regardless of where you live, fenugreek seeds and pancakes are a match made in culinary heaven. Fenugreek, the plant, is also perfect match for gardens everywhere.

FENUGREEK CARE

Fenugreek is my favorite spice to grow with kids due to its fast germination, speedy flowering, and fragrance. Soak seeds in warm water for 8 hours prior to planting. Expect germination in 2–3 days. Plant seeds ¼ inch (6 mm) deep in loamy or compost-amended soil.

Within 20–40 days, flowering starts and leads to the formation of elongated seedpods that smell like toffee candy. Seeds can be ready to harvest in as little as 70 days, but it often takes longer.

Use a legume inoculant to supercharge nitrogen fixing. Legume inoculants transmit bacteria called rhizobia to plant roots. Those bacteria convert nitrogen from the air and attach it to a plant's roots in nodules. In exchange, rhizobia convert sugars produced by the plant. With rhizobia inoculant, no additional nitrogen is needed to grow fenugreek.

Fenugreek has shallow roots. Water lightly and frequently. Once plants flower, they can tolerate some drought.

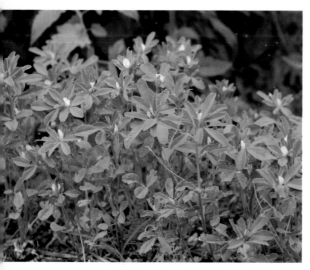

Fenugreek is a small, insubstantial plant on its own. It grows almost vinelike with small leaves and delicate flowers. Grow it as groundcover in an edible landscape or in small, densely planted patches.

Flower colors range from white to yellow and even greenish or purplish for some landrace fenugreek. White-flowered plants have larger seeds but require cool weather. Yellow-flowered varieties are more heat tolerant.

To compensate for fenugreek's spindly appearance, grow 3–4 plants in the equivalent of a square foot of soil in the ground or in a container. Or grow plants about 2–3 inches (5–7.5 cm) apart on 6-inch (15 cm) rows for peak production.

Plant fenugreek where you spend time to enjoy the fragrance.

HARVESTING

Harvest individual pods when they yellow. Or cut the entire aboveground plant at the soil line and dry it. Leave the roots in the ground so residual nitrogen remains in the soil.

Unzip the pods over a bowl, like tiny peas, while watching a sunset. Or thresh the dried pods and winnow its chaff. Expect ½ to 1 teaspoon (2.5 to 5 ml) of seeds per plant.

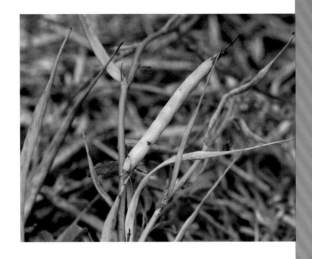

SPICE PROFILE
- **Names:** Fenugreek, Methi
- **Latin:** *Trigonella foenum-graecum*
- **Native to:** Middle East and southeastern Europe
- **Edible parts:** Leaves, seeds
- **Culinary use:** Bitter-tasting, strong maple or burnt sugar aroma, with a hint of celery that adds fragrance to curries, maple syrup substitutes, teas, and breads

GROWING CONDITIONS
- Cool-season crop; optimal seed starting 60–75°F (16–24°C); mature plant tolerance 35–90°F (2–32°C)
- Slight frost tolerance; don't overwater
- Full sun to part shade; fertile, well-draining soil; pH 6.0–8.0
- Soak seeds for 8 hours, 2–5 days to germination; 70–100 days to seed harvest
- Completely self-fertile

ABOVE: Fenugreek seedlings are small and spindly. Plant in groups for bigger impact and better weed prevention in the spice garden.

MEDICINAL TIP

Ancient Egyptians soaked fenugreek seeds in water and ground them into a paste for internal consumption and external applications.[5] The mucilaginous nature of fenugreek provides much of its medicinal actions, soothing and coating inflamed or irritated tissues. Fenugreek is used to reduce blood glucose levels and dyslipidemia in those with diabetes and insulin resistance.[6] For hyperthyroid conditions, fenugreek helps control symptoms and may potentially decrease production of thyroid hormone.[7]

MUSTARD— A MUST FOR THE SPICE GARDENER

Mustard seed is the second-most consumed spice on the planet, behind black peppercorns. Canada and Nepal are the world's top mustard producers. Despite being 68 times smaller than Canada, Nepal has even held the number one mustard production spot.

Mustard seed oil is a staple of the Nepalese diet. The raw oil is bitter and must be heated until it smokes to add the complex, savory flavor synonymous with Nepalese cooking.

In Nepal, culinary influences come from India, China, Tibet, and elsewhere. Recipes are adapted for use with available local produce and protein sources. As a result, there is a huge variety of regional cuisine styles in such a small country. Yet mustard seed, or its oil, makes it into nearly every meal.

You don't have to live in the Himalayas to cultivate a love for and an abundant supply of mustard seeds. Plant a handful of seeds into prepared soil in early spring and mustard practically grows itself.

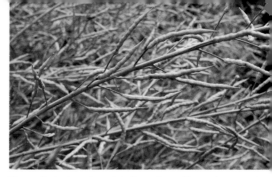

Mustard plants make a lot of seeds, so the pods grow heavy. Stake sections of plants upright or just allow room for its natural arching habit when seeding. The profusion of seedpods, in various states of drying, is even more beautiful than mustard flowers.

MUSTARD TYPES

White or yellow mustard is the variety used for hot dog mustard. It's mainly grown as a field crop and a cover crop.

Black mustard seeds have hard outer coatings that pop like popcorn when roasted. They have a strong flavor and are used for oil production and seasoning.

Leaf mustard, *Brassica juncea*, is commonly grown by home gardeners. These plants also produce large quantities of tasty brown seeds that can be used as a substitute for white, yellow, or black mustard seeds. For the home gardener, leaf mustard is most beautiful to grow and provides edible greens too.

MUSTARD CARE

Mustard can grow in poor soil, though it's more pest and disease prone. In compost-rich soil, mustard can tolerate pH ranges from 5.0–8.0. Before planting, add 3 inches (7.5 cm) of compost and incorporate a slow-release nitrogen fertilizer such as feather meal or soybean meal to the soil.

Plant seeds ¼ inch (6 mm) deep in early spring. Overseed and eat the extra seedlings as baby greens when they are 2 inches (5 cm) tall. Remaining plants need 8–10 inches (20–25 cm) of space.

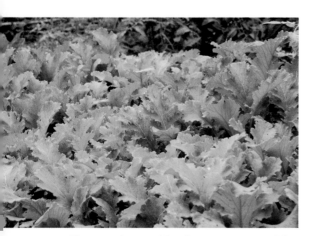

The young leaves of this *Brassica juncea* are frilly and beautiful. Plant extra and harvest the young leaves as salad greens. Grow your best seedlings into spice plants.

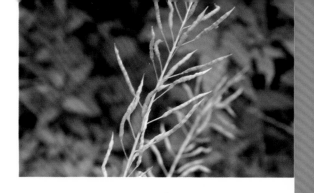

Aim for 40–60 days of growing time at temperatures between 50–75°F (13–24°C) to limit bolting. When plants begin to flower, they can grow 4–5 feet (1.2–1.5 m) tall.

Mustard can develop a 3-foot (1 m)-long taproot. Grow this spice in prepared ground, in deep raised beds, or in deep containers.

HARVESTING

Harvest before the oldest pods feel papery. Cut the seed tops just above the last leaves. Place in a paper bag, or use the candy wrapper method (see page 23), to finish drying. Thresh and remove the chaff.

Plan on 3–5 tablespoons (45–150 ml) of seeds per plant when it's planted in good soil.

MEDICINAL TIP

Mustard is known for its potent volatile oils. When used in powdered mustard seed packs or plasters, these oils create a rubefacient effect on the skin, drawing blood to the area on which the mustard is applied.[8] This circulatory stimulating activity can soothe sore muscles, reduce joint inflammation, and decrease pain as a result. Use caution as mustard can cause irritation when applied topically.[9]

ABOVE RIGHT: *Mustard seedpods put on a colorful show when drying. Colors range from green to pink, purple, yellow, and brown. Make sure to harvest before the pods begin to feel papery though, or you could end up with endlessly self-sowing mustard.*

SPICE PROFILE
- **Names:** Brown or Leaf Mustard
- **Latin:** *Brassica juncea*
- **Native to:** Cultivated worldwide
- **Edible parts:** Entire plant
- **Culinary use:** Tangy, similar to horse-radish, used in grain mustard

SPICE PROFILE
- **Names:** White or Yellow Mustard
- **Latin:** *Sinapis alba*
- **Native to:** Morocco, Europe
- **Edible parts:** Entire plant
- **Culinary use:** Mild taste used for hot dog mustard

SPICE PROFILE
- **Name:** Black Mustard
- **Latin:** *Brassica nigra*
- **Native to:** North Africa, Europe, Asia
- **Edible parts:** Entire plant
- **Culinary use:** Strong nutty flavor, seeds are cooked until they pop, also used for oil

GROWING CONDITIONS
- Cool-season crop; optimal seed starting 50–75°F (13–24°C); mature plant tolerance 28–85°F (-2–29°C)
- Some frost tolerance; susceptible to pests in heat
- Full sun to part shade; grows in most soil types; pH 5.0–8.0
- 2–5 days for seed germination; 20–40 days for leaf harvest; 100+ days to seed harvest
- Self-fertile, cross-pollination recommended

A TALE OF TWO SEEDS:
CELERY AND CARAWAY

With a little more work, you can expand your cool-season spice repertoire by growing biennials such as celery and caraway. These are grown like other cool-season annuals featured in this section. However, they require a period of *vernalization* to produce seeds.

Vernalization refers to slowing a plant's metabolism through exposure to cold. After a required number of chill hours, the plant's biological clock gives permission to flower.

Vernalization requirements vary. Caraway can flower with just 1–2 weeks of cool weather. However, for best seed production, caraway

needs 8 weeks of vernalization at around 45°F (7°C). Celery needs just 2 weeks of vernalization at 45°F (7°C) for peak production.

Not all plants that require vernalization are cold hardy. Celery only tolerates light frosts. Mature caraway can survive temperatures down to -35°F (-37°C).

After vernalization, plants still need optimal temperatures and adequate daylight hours to flower. These requirements also vary by plant. For caraway and celery, flowering happens in warm weather in late spring to early summer. Cross-pollination is also required.

Celery— *Apium graveolens*
Opt for seeds labeled as cutting, leaf, wild, smallage, or Chinese celery. These have larger seeds than stalk celery.

In winter, start seeds indoors in 8- to 12-inch-deep (15 to 30 cm) pots. Use a grow light to simulate 10 hours of daylight. When plants are several inches tall, take the pots outdoors when temperatures are between 35–45°F (2–7°C) to vernalize for 14 days total. Return pots indoors during colder weather. After the risk of frost is over, leave pots outdoors.

Grown this way, plants often produce seeds the first year. If they don't, keep them growing in pots through winter and repeat the vernalization process.

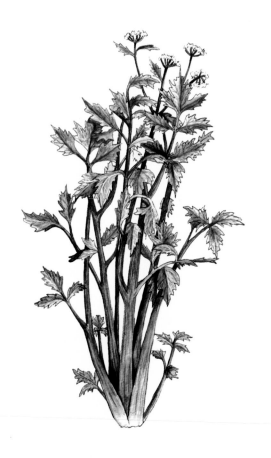

Caraway—*Carum carvi*

Plant cold-hardy caraway seeds outdoors
in cool weather in spring or a few months
before your first hard winter frost. Otherwise,
grow it like dill. For pot-grown caraway
plants, vernalize outside when temperatures
are 32–45°F (0–7°C) for at least 8 weeks.

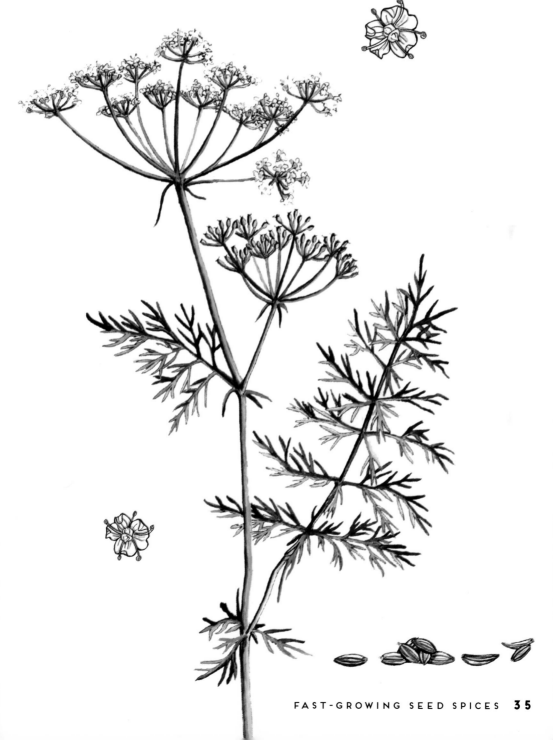

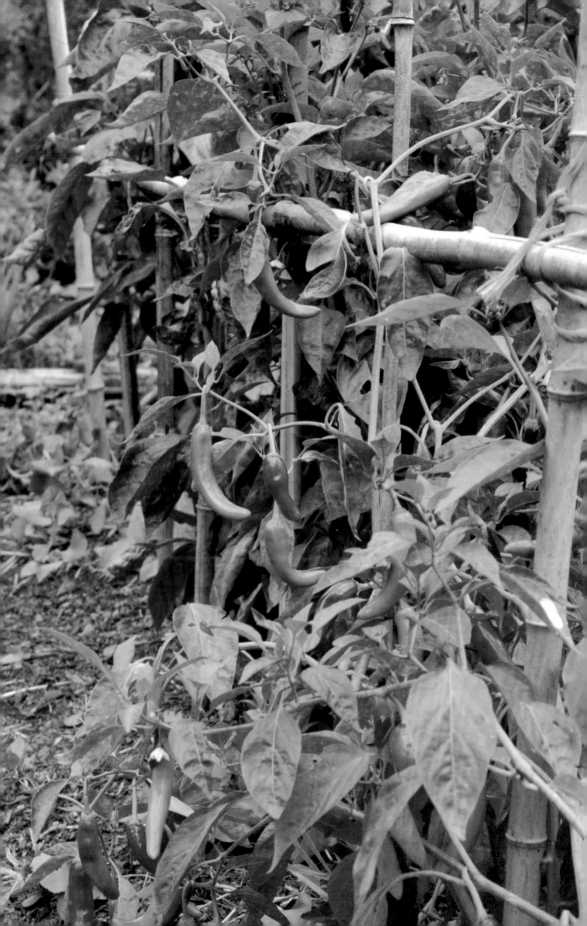

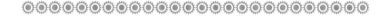

WARM-SEASON SEED SPICES

The seed spices in this section are generally started in cool weather. However, they may need a long, warm growing season for good production. Or they have better heat tolerance than the cool-season seed spices.

CUMIN	38
NIGELLA	40
SESAME	42
POPPY	44
PAPRIKA	46
SAFFRON	48

< Bamboo stakes work well for staking peppers. In windy areas or for heavy-bearing pepper varieties, connect the posts with a bamboo cross bar for added stability.

CUMIN— EXTRA CARE REQUIRED

Most of the world's cumin is produced in India and China. Cumin is difficult to produce commercially. It's grown mainly on small farms. In India, cumin is such a critical staple food, and so little is grown, the government mandated local cumin needs be met before export is allowed.

Between the complexity of growing cumin and extreme weather events, the surplus for international sales is very small. Yet the demand for cumin is increasing. Vietnam, Bangladesh, the U.S., the U.K., and others rely on the importation of cumin.

Cumin scarcity is a real risk in the future. Supply your own demand and expand your gardening skills by mastering the art of growing this spice at home.

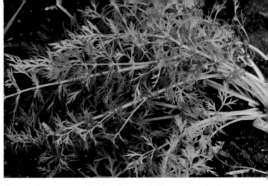

As cumin matures, its top-heavy foliage on spindly stems is subject to being knocked over by wind or rain. Contact with wet soil increases fungal risks. As plants mature, water only when the top 1–2 inches of soil feel dry to limit risks.

CUMIN CARE

Cumin is a tricky spice to grow unless you have the perfect climate. It requires a long, warm—not hot—growing season. Plants are prone to stunting and fungal pathogens in wet or humid areas. Wind tolerance is poor.

On the upside, mature cumin is drought tolerant. Plus, its compact size makes it good to grow in pots you can temporarily move indoors during inclement weather. Use individual 6-inch (15 cm) pots or grow a few plants together in larger pots.

Sow seeds indoors, in ideal conditions, 4–6 weeks before last frost. Take plants outdoors when temperatures are between 50–80°F (10–27°C) and weather is mild.

When plants bloom, leave them outdoors in a wind-protected location, near other flowers to encourage insect pollination. Grow at least three plants together for cross-pollination. Hand-pollination is ineffective.

Grow larger quantities of cumin in outdoor garden beds under the protection of low polytunnels. Temporary shade helps control temperatures on hot days. Plastic covering can protect plants in cooler or wet weather. Aim to keep plants in their sweet spot of 50–80°F (10–27°C) .

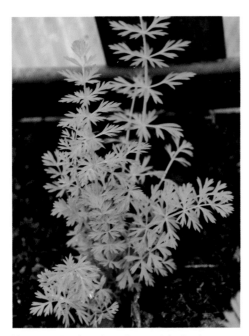

Young cumin plants have fine, upright, feathery foliage that can easily be outpaced by fast-growing weeds until the plants are nearly mature and have a significant leaf mass.

In humid areas, give plants 6-plus inches (15-plus cm) of space to limit fungal risks. In dry areas, plant 3 inches (7.5 cm) apart on 6-inch (15 cm) rows to crowd out weeds. Mulch between rows to limit weeds. Weed early and often.

To improve germination, soak seeds for 8 hours. Then sow seeds on the surface of 65°F (18°C) soil. Water deeply to settle the seeds. Mist soil with a spray bottle or misting hose twice daily until germination. Then water regularly.

Growing cumin can help you fine-tune your gardening skills. It also offers you a low risk initiation into microclimate creation using simple tools such as low tunnels and indoor seed starting.

HARVESTING

Remove seedheads when the plants begin to wither. Dry under cover. Thresh dried heads and winnow the chaff.

Plants produce about ¼–1 teaspoon of seeds each.

MEDICINAL TIP

Cumin's earthy, aromatic seed can be used medicinally to regulate insulin levels in metabolic disorders, such as insulin resistance and Type II diabetes. A research study showed the consumption of physiologically active doses of cumin seed for 8 weeks not only lowered insulin levels but resulted in considerable weight loss in overweight adults.[10] To achieve these results, you'll need more than a sprinkle in your weekly curry; larger doses of encapsulated cumin seed is recommended.

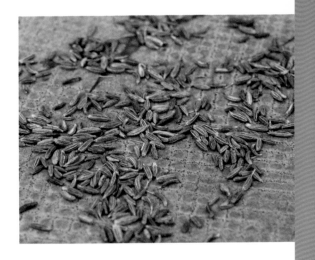

SPICE PROFILE
- **Names:** Cumin, Jeera, Zeera
- **Latin:** *Cuminum cyminum*
- **Native to:** Eastern Mediterranean, Turkestan, Egypt
- **Edible parts:** Seeds, leaves
- **Culinary use:** Musky, pungent aroma with peppery, nutty taste used in curries, pickles, breads, and to season meat

GROWING CONDITIONS
- Warm-season crop; optimal seed starting 65–80°F (18–27°C); mature plant tolerance 38–80°F (3–27°C)
- Protect from extreme heat, wind, rain, and frost
- Full sun; fertile, well-draining soil, not good for clay soil; pH 5.5–7.5
- Irregular germination; 120+ days for seed harvest
- Cross-pollination required

ABOVE: *Cumin seeds are as beautiful as they are tasty. In some cultures, they are even used like salt and pepper, sprinkled on prepared dishes to add extra flavor and texture as needed.*

NIGELLA—
BEST SUPPORTING
SPICE

Nigella is one of the most misunderstood seed spices. Frankly, until I wrote this book, I grew it for its decorative value. I didn't use my harvested seeds. Then I discovered *Panch Phoron* or Five Spice Mix.

Similar to Quatre Epice in French cooking or Chinese Five Spice, Bengali and Bangladeshi Panch Phoron is a specialty spice mix used in many recipes. When you combine equal parts fenugreek, fennel, mustard seed, cumin, and nigella—alchemical magic happens. Those first four brash spices are mellowed into a cohesive, complex base for soups, curries, and meat dishes alike.

Some other cultures understand the benefit of this beautiful supporting spice. Egyptians use it in bread or as a baked goods topping like poppy seeds. Eastern European countries have a place in their hearts and breads for Charnushka, as it is called there.

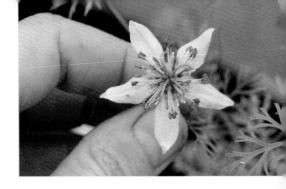

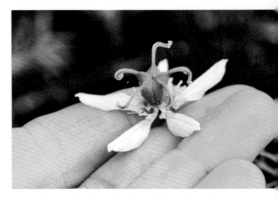

A nigella seedpod swells like a balloon from the center of its flower petals. Unpollinated pods will also start to swell, but then will desiccate and wither without forming seeds.

Unfortunately, if you live in locales where the power of a perfect supporting spice is underappreciated, nigella can be hard to find. But you'll be happy to know it's easy to grow at home!

NIGELLA CARE

Nigella sativa is related to the cottage garden favorite love-in-a-mist. The flowers are less showy and foliage spindlier than its fancier cousin. Yet when planted in groups, the effect can be lovely. Flowers range from white to pale purple or blue. Plants average 18 inches (46 cm) in height.

Nigella is easiest to grow outdoors, in spring, when temperatures will remain between 50–75°F (10–24°C) for 6–8 weeks during plant establishment. It can be fall-grown in areas with mild winters. Heat and drought tolerance increase after flowering. Too much heat or dryness before then can prevent seed set.

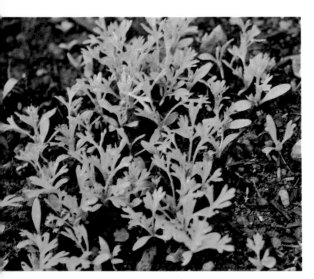

In its early stages, nigella seedlings appear similar to common weeds such as ragweed and to other spices such as coriander. They germinate irregularly so plant extra to avoid having gaps in your planting area.

Heavily overseed to ensure germination. Sow seeds on the surface of the soil and cover lightly with compost. Cover seeded areas with shade cloth or a piece of wood. Check for germination and water daily. Remove the cover when seedlings emerge.

Nigella loves soil amended with composted livestock manure. Regular compost tea applications or food-safe flower fertilizers encourage heavier bloom production.

For the best seed production, give each plant 1 square foot (.09 square meter) of space. For beauty, plant in groups on 6-inch (15 cm) centers.

HARVESTING

Harvest seedpods and dry in bags before the husks get brittle. Crack open dry pods with your hands and winnow the chaff from seeds.

Plants produce around ½ teaspoon of seeds.

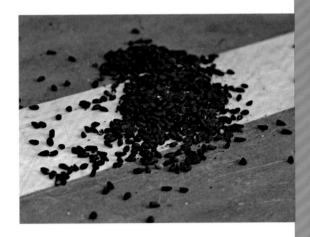

SPICE PROFILE
- **Names:** Nigella, Black Seed, Black Cumin, Fennel Flower, Kalonji, Charnushka
- **Latin:** *Nigella sativa*
- **Native to:** Most likely Western Asia, Mediterranean
- **Edible parts:** Seeds
- **Culinary use:** Mild aroma; herby, peppery, anise flavor complements breads, savory pastries, and curries

GROWING CONDITIONS
- Cool- to warm-season crop; optimal seed starting 55–70°F (13–21°C); mature plant tolerance 20–90°F (-7–32°C)
- Protect from frost in early spring; will tolerate some heat once established. Full sun; fertile, well-draining soil; pH 6.0–7.5
- Seed germination is irregular; 110–130 days for seed harvest
- Self-fertile, cross-pollination recommended

ABOVE: Nigella sativa *seeds are less well recognized than many other common seed spices. They resemble tiny, pointed splinters of charcoal. They are also called "black seed" based on their appearance. Some people confuse nigella seeds with onion or chive seeds.*

MEDICINAL TIP

Nigella has a long-standing tradition of use and is considered a panacea in its native lands. Consuming this plant's seeds has a strong protective effect on your gastrointestinal system through increased production of the mucous coating on gastric tissues. Research shows drinking a tea made from nigella seeds can reduce the formation of and reverse ulcerations through its mucus promoting activity and the plants' ability to inhibit excessive gastric acid secretion, which can be problematic in some who suffer from ulcers.[11]

SESAME— THE SURVIVAL SEED

Sesame is often called a survival plant. It tolerates extreme heat, crowding, and poor soil. There are landraces adapted to monsoon conditions and drought conditions. Sesame's fat and protein content plus its utility as an oil, paste, and flour meal have helped subsistence farmers since antiquity survive in harsh climates.

The natural dehiscence, or shattering of the seedpods, also helps ensure this plant's self-propagation. As a result, wild and naturalized sesame can be found in many warm regions of the world.

Despite 5,000 years of cultivation, industrial sesame production only became possible in the mid-1900s. A natural genetic mutation made some seedpods *indehiscent* (non-shattering). This allowed growers to breed pods that were easier to harvest mechanically. Still, sesame harvests have remained largely manual worldwide.

Dried sesame lacks the aromatic, volatile oils associated with spices. An antioxidant called sesamol prevents its oils from volatizing. Sesame is even used to make margarine and ghee shelf-stable. Yet once the seeds are roasted or toasted, all that oil volatility activates, revealing sesame's spicy

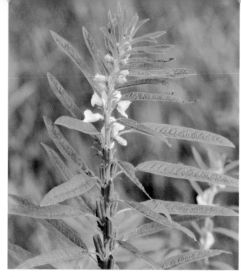

Sesame plants and flowers are quite beautiful. The pods are ready to pick when they are mostly dry.

nature. In other words, cooking causes the flavor to . . . *open sesame*. (You had to see that one coming!)

Sesame plants benefit the soil. They reduce the numbers of harmful nematodes and fungal pathogens. Its pervasive root structure breaks up soil compaction. Sesame is also beautiful in pollinator and bird gardens. It grows 2–6 feet (61 cm–2m) tall, with bell-shaped flowers that open for weeks.

SESAME CARE

Sesame requires temperatures above 70°F (21°C) for good growth. Some sesame varieties tolerate wet conditions while others only thrive in dry conditions.

Commercial white sesame seeds are hulled. The black seeds, prized by gastronomes, have edible hulls. There is also a range of colors between black and white to grow in home gardens.

In consistently hot weather seedpods are harvestable in about 90 days. Otherwise, plan on harvesting between 110–130 days.

For an early start, plant seeds indoors 6–8 weeks before ideal outdoor conditions. Use an electric seed mat to warm the soil. Sow seeds ¼ inch (6 mm) deep. Water daily until germination.

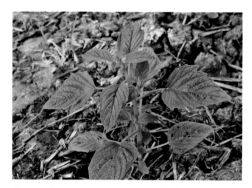

Sesame is an easy-to-grow spice that produces mature seeds in about 3–4 months.

Plant outdoors when temperatures are consistently above 70°F (21°C). Use row covers and mulch to keep the soil warm.

Some sesame grows in a narrow, nonbranching fashion suited to rows. Others are branching and require more space. Some varieties need dense planting for production; others need more space.

Incorporate 3–4 inches (7.5–10 cm) of compost into soil before planting. Add feather meal, bat guano, or other slow-release nitrogen sources for the best yields.

HARVESTING

For small production, pick individual pods when they are mostly dry. Finish drying on a baking sheet or drying rack. Let the plants continue to grow. Like okra, pods will keep forming at the top of a plant.

For larger harvests, when 75 percent of the lower pods show signs of drying, cut the tops. Hang-dry the heads in a paper bag or dry on a tarp to minimize losses. Thresh and winnow the chaff.

Expect 1–3 tablespoons (15–45 ml) of seeds per plant.

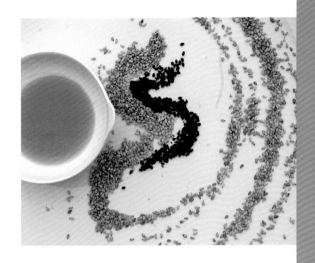

SPICE PROFILE

- **Names:** Sesame, Benne, Beni, Benni
- **Latin:** *Sesamum indicum*
- **Native to:** Probably India
- **Edible parts:** Seeds
- **Culinary use:** Oily, nutty flavor well suited to toasting; used in savory dishes, breads, candy, pastry, and tahini

GROWING CONDITIONS

- Warm-season crop; optimal seed starting 70–85°F (21–29°C); mature plant tolerance 55–105°F (13–40.5°C)
- Protect from soil temperatures below 65°F (18°C)
- Full sun; fertile, well-draining soil; pH 5.5–7.5
- 2–5 days for seed germination; 90–130 to seed harvest
- Self-fertile, cross-pollination recommended

ABOVE: *Store-bought sesame seeds are typically all white because they are hulled and sorted for color purity. At home, you can grow sesame in a range of colors. To hull seeds, soak them in warm water overnight, then rub off the hulls and sort the seeds. Or just eat the seeds in their delicious hulls.*

MEDICINAL TIP

The seeds of sesame provide a rich medicine. The oil, abundant in lignans and tocopherols, demonstrates prolific antioxidant activity.[12] Consumption of the seeds may reduce blood pressure through the beneficial lipid content, shown to decrease the narrowing of the arteries and oxidative damage.[13] Sprinkle the seeds liberally on foods or eat more tahini for these favorable effects.

POPPY SEEDS—
FOR REMEMBRANCE

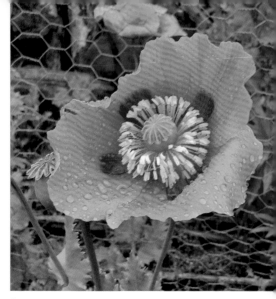

Stunning poppy flowers give way to round pods that swell with seeds.

I have to warn you—in some places growing poppies is illegal or at least controversial. The poppy varieties that produce edible seeds also make opium. Opium is used in prescription pharmaceuticals and illegal drug production. It's at the heart of our global opioid epidemic.

Unfortunately, in some troubled parts of the world, growing illicit poppies is the only way small farmers survive. It's troubling to think about the global disparities in freedom of choice. Yet it's very important to acknowledge that they exist, as doing so leads to greater compassion.

I grow poppies to remind me there's more to the story than seen in media glimpses or vacations.

Incidentally, corn poppies (*Papaver rhoeas*), cousin to breadseed poppies, appeared in war fields near WWI mass cemeteries in Belgium. The scene of endless red poppies emerging in that disturbed soil was so moving, it inspired poetry, and of wearing red poppies as a sign of remembrance.

I can't advise you on the legality of growing seed poppies. However, many poppy laws factor in a gardener's intent when growing them. If your reasons are beauty, seeds, and as a meditation to open your heart to greater understanding of other cultures—unless law enforcement has reason to doubt your integrity—there's a good chance you can grow them legally.

POPPY CARE

The most productive poppies for seeds typically have "breadseed" in the variety name. However, any poppy that starts with *Papaver somniferum* var. *XYZ* will produce delicious seeds. Feel free to choose decorative *Papaver somniferum* varieties for your flower garden and your spice rack.

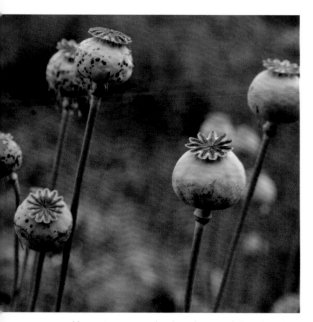

Harvest poppy pods when they are fully colored but before the vents open if you don't want any accidental seeding. Clip the stems well below the pods, collect multiple stems together with a rubber band, and set inside a paper bag to finish drying.

Poppies grow best outdoors when planted in the ground with minimal care. A couple of weeks before your area's last frost, spread a handful of poppy seeds over an area with good garden soil. Water lightly every few days until plants emerge. Then water regularly. When plants are 2 inches (5 cm) tall, cut extra seedlings at the soil level.

You can also grow poppies in deep, wide pots or raised planter beds. Potted poppies need weekly compost tea or slow-release flower fertilizer. Poppies grown in compost-amended garden soil usually don't need fertilizer.

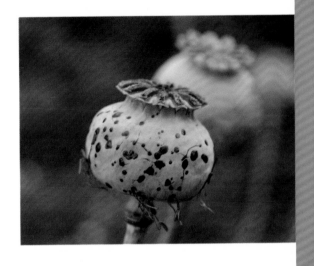

HARVESTING

Flowers give way to a round seedpod with a flat, starlike top. The pod swells, then stalls, and eventually begins to dry in various Easter egg hues. Once dry, vents open below the star's lid. Pour the seeds through the vents into a jar to harvest.

For some decorative varieties, or for pods dried off the plant, vents don't always open. In that case, when the pod sounds like a baby's rattle, pry the flat top off and pour the seeds out.

Production varies by variety from a quarter teaspoon to ½–2 tablespoons (7.5–30 ml) per plant.

SPICE PROFILE
- **Names:** Poppy, Breadseed Poppy, Opium Poppy
- **Latin:** *Papaver somniferum*
- **Native to:** southwestern Asia, Mediterranean
- **Edible parts:** Seeds
- **Culinary use:** Nutty, oily, sweet-enhancing flavor used in baked goods, desserts, salad dressings, and oil production

GROWING CONDITIONS
- Cool- to warm-season crop; optimal seed starting 50–65°F (10–18°C); mature plant tolerance 28–85°F (-2–29°C)
- Protect from extreme heat until pods form
- Full sun; fertile, well-draining soil; pH 6.5–7.5
- Irregular germination; 100–120 days for seed harvest
- Partially self-fertile, cross-pollination recommended

ABOVE: *Poppy seedpods are as beautiful as the flowers. They come in Easter egg colors, with a star top and triangular vents just below the flat top that expand and open as the pod dries until the seeds simply pour out through the vents.*

PAPRIKA, PIMENTÓN, AND GOCHU— POTENT POWERHOUSES

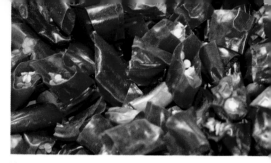

Most peppers or chilies are native to the Americas. They found their way to Europe through the Spanish and Portuguese spice trades and spread globally from there.

In Europe, new varieties such as Hungarian paprika or Spanish pimentón (dulce, agridulce, or picante) were bred to suit the subtle preferences of dill-, fennel-, and saffron-favoring palates. In Asian countries, hotter varieties were embraced and propagated.

Likewise, the popular Korean gochu pepper used in kimchi was long believed to have been introduced as a result of these spice trades. However, Korean researchers challenge this notion. They make a compelling case that the taste profile, Scoville rating (capsaicin measure), and nutritional aspects of gochu distinguish it from other *Capsicum annum* varieties. They also refer to ancient writings that reference gochu before it could have been imported to the Korean Peninsula.

Peppers used for making spice have thicker skins and less flesh than peppers for eating fresh. They dry faster and are less rot-prone. Plants tend to be highly productive.

Cultivar descriptions that reference paprika, pimentón, or gochu are a great place to start your spice production from peppers.

Use scissors to cut your dried peppers into pieces that will easily fit into a spice grinder. If you want to remove the seeds, cut peppers in half lengthwise. Scrape out the seeds and cut to size.

PEPPER CARE

Plant seeds ¼ inch (6 mm) deep in warm conditions, around the first day of spring. In climates with long, hot growing seasons, you can direct plant outdoors. Otherwise, start seeds indoors.

For indoor seed starting, warming mats shorten germination. Give seedlings plenty of light to prevent them from becoming leggy. Transplant outdoors when daytime and evening temperatures are above 70°F (21°C) and 45°F (7°C) respectively.

Plant seedlings deeper than the original plant root depth to create a more deeply rooted plant. Burying the lower section of stem encourages *adventitious* root development, which better anchors pepper plants. Adventitious roots start on the stem and become true roots upon contact with soil.

Space plants 8–12 inches (20–25 cm) apart. Keep sweet peppers at least 200 feet (61 m) away from hot peppers to avoid flavor muddling. Muddling occurs in the first generation because it alters the seed and spice taste. So a powdered sweet paprika could taste hot.

Tie your pepper plant loosely to a stake. Or use a cage appropriate to your plant's expected mature size. Drying peppers also grow well in containers at least 1 gallon (3.8 L) in size.

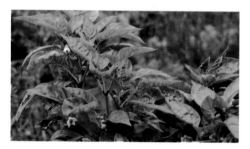

Abundant star-shaped paprika flowers give way to tiny fruits that develop quickly into large peppers. However, it can take weeks after mature size is reached before the peppers color and begin to dry.

HARVESTING

Drying peppers are ready to harvest when they turn their final color and the skin shows signs of desiccation.

Remove peppers from the plant. Use a needle and thread to sew the peppers together in a strand. Direct the needle through the colored body of the pepper rather than the green tops since the dried tops sometimes separate from the skins. Then hang in a dry shaded area, or dry them on racks in a dehydrator.

PROCESSING

Wear a mask and gloves. Work in a well-ventilated space. For deeper color and milder flavor, remove the seeds. Discard any discolored or moldy peppers.

Cut the dried peppers into 1-inch (2.5 cm) pieces to fit in your spice grinder. For gochugaru (Korean pepper flakes), aim for a mix of small pieces and powder. For paprika and pimentón, grind until it's finely powdered.

Expect about 1 pint (.5 L) of powder for every 1–2 pepper plants.

MEDICINAL TIP

The burning, heated sensation one receives on consumption of chili peppers alerts us to the capsaicin content and the presence of this pungent medicine. The capsaicin molecule is a blood mover, stimulating circulation and increasing vasodilation. Capsaicin-containing plants can inhibit the transmission of pain, while reducing inflammation, making it a great topical application to nerve pain, sore muscles, and joints.[14] Eat often or use in the form of a cream, compress, or soak.

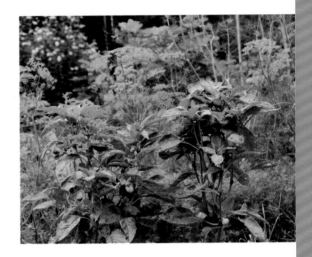

SPICE PROFILE
- **Names:** Paprika, Pimentón, Gochu, Peppers, Chillies, Chilies, Chili Peppers
- **Latin:** *Capsicum annuum*
- **Native to:** The Americas and possibly Korea
- **Edible parts:** Fruits including seeds
- **Culinary use:** Sweet, savory, and/or fiery used to flavor hearty dishes, sausages, ferments, and more

GROWING CONDITIONS
- Warm-season crop; optimal seed starting 70–85°F (21–29°C); mature plant tolerance 38–105°F (3–41°C)
- Protect from frost, freezing, and extended cool weather
- Full sun; fertile, well-draining soil; pH 6.0–7.5
- 3–14 days for seed germination; 85+ days for fruit harvest
- Completely self-fertile

ABOVE: *Peppers are a perfect companion to most of your garden herbs, spices, and vegetables. They produce for several months and can be transplanted just in time to bring color and beauty when your cool-season spices are ready to harvest. For example, as dill is setting seed, a paprika plant is beginning to produce.*

SAFFRON—
A TRULY SEASONAL SPICE

Saffron (*Crocus sativus*) is a fall-grown crocus started from a corm (a bulb-like structure). Planting corms is very much like planting seed spices, only the planting depth is much deeper. Also, instead of collecting seeds, you'll hand-harvest three stigmas from each newly opened flower.

Each corm produces 3–6 flowers, or 9–18 stigmas (which are called *threads* once dried). Stigmas are dried in a cool, dark location. Threads are stored in a small container for several months prior to use to increase aroma.

Saffron corms are triggered to grow by waning day length and cooling soil temperatures. As such, they only grow well in climates with noticeable seasonal changes from summer to fall.

Also, after flowering, plants need up to 6 months of mild conditions to produce new corms. Plants are cold hardy to 15°F (-9°C) (or a bit colder with heavy mulching). However, overall average temperatures should be between 30–65°F (-1–18°C) for peak corm production.

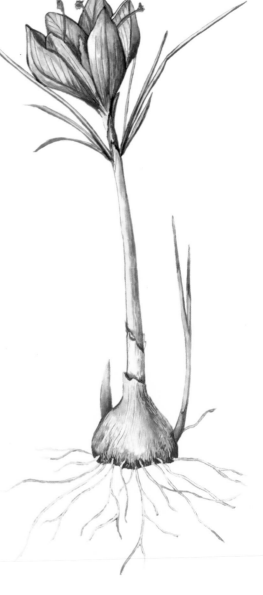

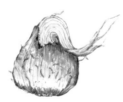

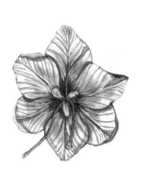

In ideal conditions, each parent corm will produce several new corms each year. Every 3 years dig up the corms, divide them, and replant in a new location to increase your harvest. Dispose of diseased corms.

You can also buy corms yearly and grow saffron as an annual. It's more costly than buying saffron, but it's fun to try.

Starting Saffron

About 6–8 weeks before outdoor soil temperatures begin to drop, plant 1-inch (or larger) corms pointy end up, 5–6 inches (12.7–15 cm) deep in the soil. Plant on 6-inch (15 cm) diameters or 4 inches (10 cm) apart on 8-inch (20 cm) rows.

Soil should be at least 10–12 inches (20–25 cm) deep with 5 percent organic matter for best corm production. Also, apply a slow-release fertilizer with some nitrogen, more phosphorus, and a little potassium (e.g., 4-5-3) monthly. Amend soil with calcium if it's depleted.

Raised beds or large outdoor pots can be used too. In cold climates, after flowering, pots could be moved to a sunny indoor location with ideal temperatures to keep growing leaves for corm production.

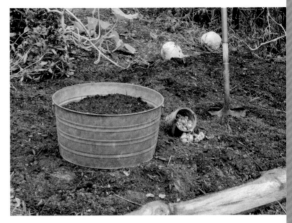
Deep soil and the addition of compost are critical to saffron production.

Water deeply upon planting and every 2 weeks thereafter until flowers emerge. After flowering, water only when the soil is dry more than 2 inches (5 cm) deep to limit disease risks.

When the tops die back, you can plant short-season, shallow-rooted plants as filler in your saffron bed. Make sure to clear out crops, add compost, and fertilize in midsummer to prepare for a second season of saffron.

MEDICINAL TIP

The beautiful stigmas of saffron hold potent antidepressant and neural anti-inflammatory effects[15] capable of uplifting people's moods and reducing inflammation in the brain. Take a few stigmas and make a crimson cup of tea to get the benefits of this spice.

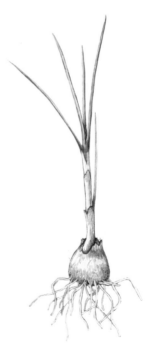

SECTION 2
THE SPICE UNDERGROUND

In the previous section we covered planting spices from and for seeds. If you are comfortable with those skills, then you are ready to grow horseradish, ginger, galangal, wasabi, and more. Growing underground spices requires the same basic skills as growing seed spices with four notable differences.

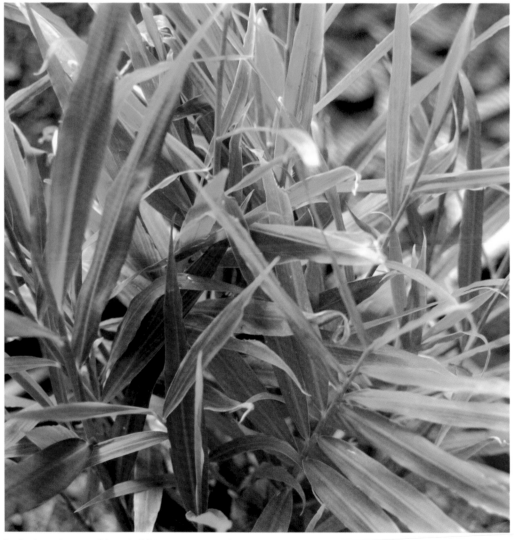

Lush ginger leaves add tropical flair to a spice garden.

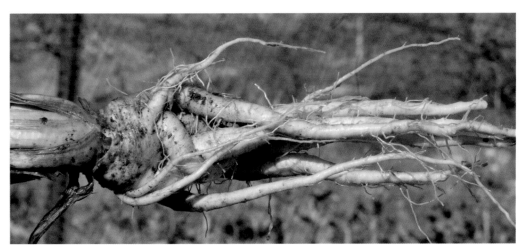

Roots are amazingly adaptive. This taprooted chicory became fibrous in dense clay soil. It may not be a perfect chicory specimen, yet it will still make a tasty coffee alternative.

First, in some cases you may sow root cuttings or rhizome pieces instead of seeds. Ginger, for example, is grown by placing a portion of a rhizome (a chunky, rootlike structure) in soil. Horseradish is grown from a root cutting. Wasabi is grown from seed or plantlets that form from its enlarged stem.

Second, when growing plants for their underground parts, you need deep, well-draining soil for ideal production. Soil like that can take years of preparation to achieve in the ground. Fortunately, all the spices in this section can be planted in soil mixes in containers or raised beds.

Third, you don't harvest the aboveground plant parts as spice. Instead, you carefully dig out your spice crops from the depths of your soil and clean them prior to processing.

Finally, there are some post-harvest differences. Harvested garlic needs to be *cured*. Ginger can be used fresh or sliced, dried, and powdered. Horseradish is grated and preserved in vinegar. These methods are no more difficult than seed processing. They just require know-how.

Our first underground spice—chicory—is used to spice up coffee or act as a coffee substitute.

Some spice hardliners may not even consider it a spice. I think chicory counts because the mature harvested root is used as a water-soluble flavoring agent and not for its caloric content. Additionally, it has a distinct aroma.

I also included it because if you are new to growing spices for underground parts, chicory is totally groundbreaking. I mean that literally. It can help break up soil compaction in your garden. That makes it a perfect gateway spice to transition your garden from growing spices for seeds to growing spices for their underground parts.

Likewise, growing the other plants in this section is also the perfect gateway to help you further develop your skills as a gardener. Most people start gardening by thinking about everything above the ground such as pests, weather, and plant appearance. When you grow roots, rhizomes, and other underground spices, you begin to see beneath the surface to all the hidden complexities at play in producing healthy plants.

Let's dig deeper to unearth the spice secrets growing beneath the soil.

TECHNIQUES FOR GROWING ROOTS, BULBS, AND RHIZOMES

Most roots come in two forms: fibrous and taprooted. Fibrous roots grow Medusa-like under the crown of a plant. Taproots grow one central root with branching side roots resembling an upside-down tree. Some plants start with a taproot and then develop fibrous roots. Damaged taproots may become fibrous to compensate. Some plants even have aboveground aerial roots that we'll cover in section three.

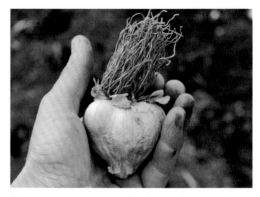

This garlic head is made of multiple individual bulbs, often called cloves, that can each become a plant in the right conditions. Below the head is a fibrous root system.

STORAGE ROOT

The basic function of a root, regardless of how it grows, is to gather nutrients and water. However, several plants have evolved roots that do more than seek life-sustaining inputs. They also store large quantities of nutrients for later use. Plants with taproots such as chicory, horseradish, and licorice fall into this category. In those cases, the part we use as spice is a fattened underground taproot.

Taprooted plants can often be grown from seed. However, some are easier to start using a portion of the root called a cutting. The root is not the primary reproductive organ of these plants. Yet like a lizard that regrows a lost tail, a cutting can regrow the missing parts of the plant.

Think about how incredible that is. A small piece of a root that spent its life underground can be cut away from the rest of its plant body. Replanted, it will reliably reconstruct the other 95 percent of itself using nothing but good soil, water, and sunlight. It's like a 3D printer that makes its own CAD plans, sources the thermoplastics, and operates without electricity.

BULBS

The edible portion of garlic is not a root at all; it's a divided bulb. A bulb also stores nutrients and water. However, it stores them in the fattened underground stem of the plant. Fibrous roots that grow below the bulb collect nutrients and water. Then the roots transfer them up to the stem. The stem stores any excess nutrients in bulbs.

Bulbs aren't just storage devices, though. They're primary reproductive mechanisms. When a bulb reaches its maximum nutrient-holding capacity, it splits into a second bulb, and a third, and so on as necessary to store nutrients. In garlic, we call the divided bulbs cloves.

Each clove, in the right environmental conditions, will grow roots and sprout greens, and become a full-fledged plant. Then that plant will begin making bulbs of its own.

RHIZOMES

Rhizomes, such as the harvested parts of ginger and turmeric, are also modified underground stems that store nutrients. However, rather than making a series of bulbs in one place, nutrient-fattened rhizomes spread out laterally in the soil.

When environmental conditions are right, nodes form on the rhizomes. On an aboveground plant stem, nodes produce leaves and branches. Underground, that node first fattens into what is often called an eye when it's seen on harvested rhizomes. Then it grows its own roots and shoots. As those roots and shoots gather nutrients, the node expands into a rhizome and begins to store excess nutrients.

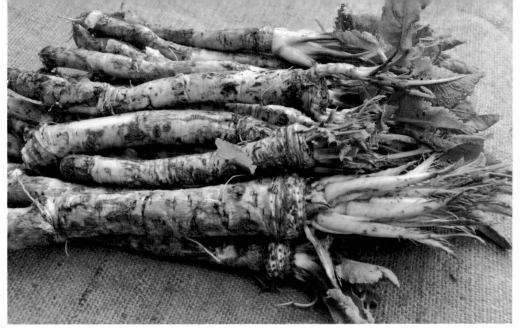

The long, thick taproots of horseradish plants break through the soil, but a planting site with deep, rich soil gets the plants off to a good start.

Rhizomes are also the primary reproductive mechanism for some plants. This is why we start some plants such as ginger by using a portion of the mature rhizome.

ENLARGED STEM

Wasabi is a special case. The nutrient-storage portion of the plant is a fattened stem similar to a rhizome, but it grows vertically like a taproot. Wasabi also produces nodes and new plants similar to a rhizome. However, it makes them on the plant's crown at the soil surface, not underground. These baby plants are called *plantlets*.

In retail, wasabi sold for spice is often called a rhizome. In gardening literature, the spice portion is typically called an enlarged stem. Regardless of what you call it, most people have never tasted real wasabi. That's because wasabi is a bit tricky to grow, extremely expensive, and best used fresh. Most retail products labeled as wasabi are a horseradish and mustard mix dyed green.

In all these cases, humans take advantage of these natural plant storage and reproductive modifications by harvesting them for our own

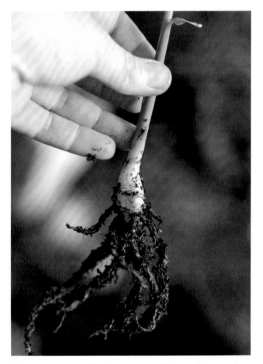

This ginger eye, which was started from a rhizome, has its own fibrous root system. In ideal conditions, after about 10 months of growing time, this tiny plant can create its own large ginger rhizome for you to harvest. Or you can eat this entire baby ginger plant fresh—leaves, shoots, eyes, and roots—chopped up in salads.

use. To get the biggest harvests possible, though, we need to provide ideal conditions for their underground production.

GROWING TAPROOTS

True taprooted spices are soil breakers. Their nature is to grow downward to search and store nutrients and water that get washed deep in the soil.

Taproots send out tiny side roots as they grow. If those side roots find too many nutrients in the top few inches of soil and none deeper down, the taproot remains where the nutrients are. Also, if soil isn't deep enough, taproots fork into fibrous-appearing roots that only fatten a little.

To encourage long and large storage taproots to use for spice, you need soil that is 12–18 inches (30–46 cm) deep. That soil must also be very well draining so that nutrients and water flow deep into the soil rather than sitting in the top few inches.

GROWING BULBS

Bulbs have fibrous root systems growing below the bulb level. Those roots behave similar to stringy mopheads. When pressed against a hard floor, the mop strands flatten out in all directions. When dipped in a deep bucket of water, the strands float down and all around. Similarly, fibrous roots spread wide in shallow soil with a hardpan bottom. Or they flow deeper in loose soil.

Bulbs can grow in shallower soil if they have a wide area for roots to spread. However, soil that is well draining on top and hardpan below is subject to becoming boggy. Because an underground bulb is a part of the stem, it will rot in excess moisture just as an aboveground stem would.

Bulbs grow best, with less risk of rot, in soil that is at least 10–12 inches (25–30 cm) deep, well draining, with fertilizing targeted to the root zone rather than the bulb area.

Additionally, water deeply and less frequently. Allow the top couple inches of soil to dry, but don't let it crust between waterings.

GROWING RHIZOMES

Rhizomes are like bulbs that expand sideways, like a hand laid flat. As such, they need the same deep soil and nutrients. They require good drainage to keep rhizomes from rotting just like bulbs do. But they also need extra-loose soil so those rhizome bodies can expand in all directions.

Looser soil—often made by incorporating things such as coconut coir, peat moss, vermiculite, or leaf mold—drains very fast. So rhizomes in the right soil need more frequent watering to keep roots from drying out.

Finally, rhizomes tend to be what we call heavy feeders—meaning that they need more nutrients than taproots and bulbs for good rhizome production.

Extra fertility, deep, loose, well-draining soil, and lots of room for rhizomes to spread is required for plants such as ginger, galangal, turmeric, and cardamom.

Now, with cardamom, we don't eat the rhizomes. (Though they smell amazing and might be edible.) But I've included it in this underground spice section because to get a good harvest of cardamom pods, you'll need to care for it like the plants we do harvest for rhizomes. Also, cardamom makes a nice transition from underground spices to perennial spices since it takes 3 years, or more, to produce.

FERTILIZING STRATEGIES UNDERGROUND SPICES

Here are a few strategies to help you get fertilizer in the right place for growing healthy underground spices.

General Fertilizing

- Avoid top applications of fertilizer immediately before planting. Instead spread fertilizer such as composted chicken or other manures early (e.g., in late winter for early spring planting) so that precipitation and soil life will move nutrients deeper into the soil.
- Incorporate any last-minute applied fertilizers several inches deep into the soil.
- During the growing season, use water-soluble fertilizers such as compost tea applied less frequently, but with heavier dilution (e.g., 15:1 water to compost tea) so nutrients percolate deep.

For Bulbs

- Dig 4- to 6-inch (10–15 cm)-deep trenches between plant rows. Add fertilizer and cover again with soil. Plants bulbs a few inches away from the trench on either side. Roots will reach into the trench as needed for nutrients. Water the trench when you water the plants to help disperse nutrients.
- For commercial fertilizer, choose one that is phosphorous heavy to put in your trench. Or use chicken manure or worm castings as organic fertilizer and add bonemeal or green sand to increase phosphorous rates.

For Taproots

- If your soil has residual fertility from earlier grown crops, don't fertilize at all. Let the plant roots dig deep and glean those nutrients that washed into the lower levels.
- Otherwise, general fertilizing rules apply.

For Rhizomes

- Rhizomes, like bulbs, benefit from extra phosphorous such as bonemeal or soft rock phosphate when planted. Incorporate it into the soil below where the rhizome is planted.
- Incorporate slow-release nitrogen fertilizer such as feather meal, bat guano, or other sources into the top 2 inches (5 cm) of soil every 4 weeks during the growing season and water in.
- Consistent levels of potassium is also necessary for rhizome production. Compost may contain enough potassium, but if more is needed then green sand or kelp are good organic sources.
- For rhizomes that need a winter dormancy period, stop fertilizer applications in cool weather.

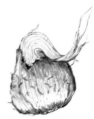

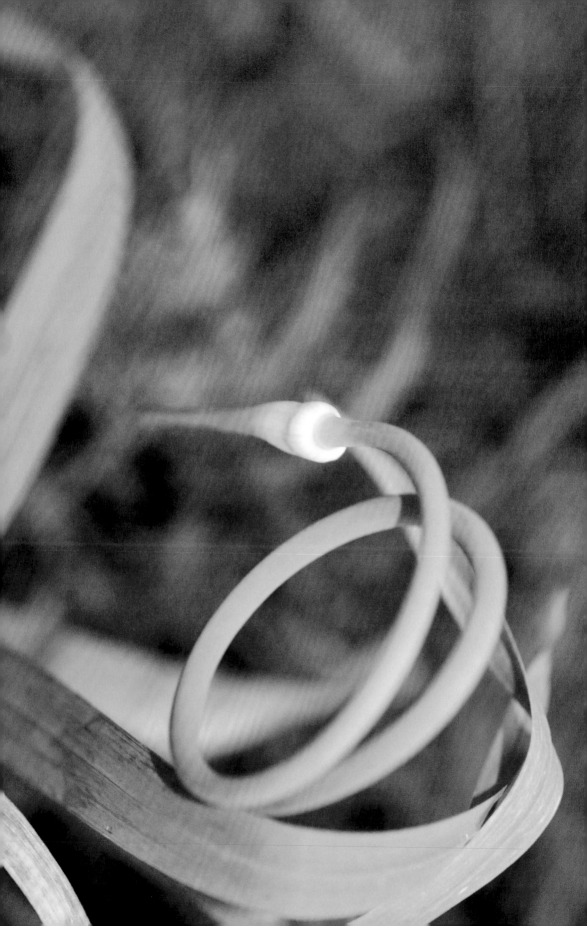

TEMPERATE CLIMATE SPICES

These underground spices like cool conditions and may need extra protection during extended warm periods.

CHICORY	58
HORSERADISH	60
GARLIC	62
LICORICE	64

< Garlic scapes are flowers that grow from hardneck garlic plants. They can be cut to the start of the stem, above the leafy tops. Sauté them or chop them raw for use in salads. Even non-garlic lovers enjoy their savory-sweet taste. Garlic heads are ready to harvest shortly after these scapes appear.

CHICORY ROOT—
FOR SELF-SUFFICIENT
COFFEE DRINKERS

Chicory has been used medicinally and as a food source since ancient times. Its application as a beverage likely began in Holland. However, its popularity as a coffee substitute occurred under the reign of Napoleon Bonaparte. Growing chicory was meant to decrease French dependence on colonial luxury products such as coffee.

The raw roots are extremely bitter and would be considered inedible by many. Yet, once dried and roasted, they develop a smoky, chocolaty, and yes . . . coffeelike flavor. Chicory powder, infused in hot water, exudes deep, rich brown color with a hearty mouthfeel.

Chicory doesn't offer the same stimulant properties as a cup of Joe. Still, if you want a satisfying, coffeelike beverage without caffeine, chicory is perfect. Or you can extend your coffee budget by mixing bought beans with homegrown chicory to make what's become known as New Orleans-style coffee.

Also try simmering your powdered chicory Turkish-style with a few cardamom pods and sugar. Then serve, unfiltered, in demitasse cups as an after-dinner drink or decaf alternative.

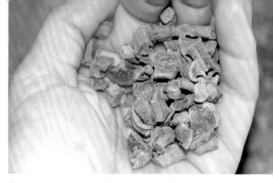

Cut, dry, and roast coffee bean-sized pieces of chicory. Then store in a recycled coffee bean bag or jar in your pantry. You can take chicory beans out as needed and grind them fresh in your coffee grinder.

CHICORY CARE

Ideally, opt for seeds cultivated for root production (*Cichorium intybus* var. *sativum*). These cultivars grow thick like parsnips or sugar beets.

Mix a slow-release nitrogen source such as feather or alfalfa meal deep into the soil prior to planting. Plant seeds ¼ inch (6 mm) deep in prepared ground or in 18- to 36-inch (46–91 cm)-deep raised beds or pots. Water twice weekly until germination; then water as needed.

In temperate climates, plant in early spring, just before the last expected frost. In hot climates, start seeds in late summer and grow from fall to spring.

Commercially, chicory is planted 6 inches apart. At home, I scatter seeds to plant. Then I thin to the best 4–5 chicory roots per square foot (.09 m²). These roots don't seem to mind crowding.

SOIL BREAKING

You can also plant chicory in poor soil with no additional nitrogen. Till the top 2–4 inches (5–10 cm) of soil before planting seeds. Roots will be slower to establish and harder to harvest. However, they will help drive organic matter and beneficial soil life deeper into the ground, making the soil easier to work in the future.

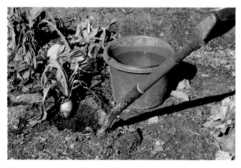

As you harvest, put roots directly into a bucket of water to rinse and keep the skins from hardening. Then you won't need to peel them to make chicory beans as a coffee substitute. As soon as you finish harvesting, rinse the roots and scrub gently to prepare them for further processing.

PREVENT FLOWERING

Chicory usually requires vernalization to flower. However, extended heat can trigger first-year flowering. If a plant begins to flower, cut the greens to the root top. Then mulch and water regularly through warm weather to keep the soil cool. Or harvest early and use the small roots.

HARVESTING

In cool climates, harvest roots in fall or winter after a few frosts, but before a hard freeze. In hot climates, harvest in spring before the heat sets in.

Use a deep spade or digging fork to loosen soil then remove the entire root.

PROCESSING

Cut roots into coffee bean-sized pieces. Dry on baking pans for 1–2 days. Then, roast in the oven on 250° (120°C or gas mark ½) until the pieces turn warm brown all over. Roasting time varies by moisture content. Turn pieces to roast both sides evenly. Lower the heat if any burning occurs before browning is complete.

Cool completely. Then grind as you would coffee until it's powdery fine.

MEDICINAL TIP

Chicory root is bitter and nutritive. Containing high amounts of the prebiotic inulin, it feeds the beneficial bacteria in your intestines, bestowing wide-ranging physiological effects such as increased digestion and metabolism.[16] A hepatoprotective plant, chicory is used to promote liver health through reduction of oxidative damage.[17] Why not treat your liver and gut microbiome to a tasty, health-promoting cup of roasted chicory root instead of coffee?

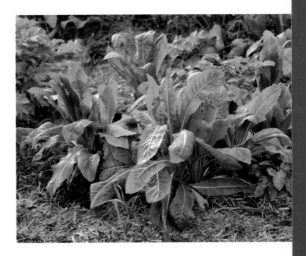

SPICE PROFILE
- **Names:** Coffee chicory, Endive, Coffeeweed
- **Latin:** *Cichorium intybus* (var. *sativum*)
- **Native to:** Europe
- **Edible parts:** Entire plant
- **Culinary use:** Bitter and peppery raw; sweet-smelling and less bitter roasted; used as a coffee additive or substitute.

GROWING CONDITIONS
- Cool-season perennial, grown as an annual
- Optimal seed starting 50–65°F (10–18°C); mature plant tolerance -30–85°F (-1–29°C)
- Protect from heat and prevent flowering
- Full sun; fertile, well-draining soil; pH 5.5–7.5
- Irregular germination; 120–180 days for large roots

ABOVE: *Chicory greens mature quickly and are quite beautiful when mulched and kept lush with regular watering. I grow chicory in my potato beds since that soil is perfect for deep-rooted plants. Sometimes an unharvested potato sprouts in with my chicory greens.*

HORSERADISH— ROOTS THAT ROAM

When excavated fresh from the soil, horseradish has no aroma. Until you break its skin, you would never know the potency inside. Once you do, enzymes exposed to air volatize and create the nose-clearing "burn" commonly associated with horseradish.

That potency quickly mellows unless you preserve horseradish in vinegar. The standard 5 percent acidity of distilled vinegar has a neutral flavor and works well for this. Just smash freshly grated horseradish into a jar and fully submerge it in vinegar as fast as you can. Or cut up pieces and put them in your food processor, pulse to perfection, add vinegar, and jar.

The trick is to stop the air exposure by adding vinegar exactly when the freshly grated horseradish tastes perfect to you. Generally, that will be between 30 seconds to a few minutes of breaking its skin.

Growing horseradish is as easy as preserving it if you know its secrets. Frankly, few people take the time to fully appreciate the features that make horseradish one of the most fascinating spices to grow.

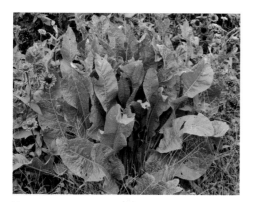

You can grow annual crops adjacent to deeply rooted horseradish. I like to pair my horseradish with zinnias or basil. Those shallow-rooted annuals help shade the soil and keep the deeper horseradish roots cool even in my hot southern climate.

In deep, fertile soil it develops a thick, straight taproot. At whatever depth the soil becomes nutrient-depleted or compacted, the root turns at a 90-degree angle. Then that root grows horizontally until it reaches soil with more nutrients. From there it grows downward again, until the nutrients run out and it makes another turn.

Plant stress, or severing, will cause parts of those pervasive roots to send stems skyward. There, they form a crown and leaves and become a new plant.

This capacity to seek ever-deeper soil and to reproduce when injured or threatened lead some people to call horseradish "invasive." As a horseradish lover, I just call it "easy to grow." Still, if you want your horseradish to stay in place, grow it in a deep, elevated container.

HORSERADISH CARE

Start horseradish several weeks before last frost, as soon as you can work the soil. Space in-ground plants, grown as an annual, 2–3 feet (61–91 cm) apart. Or use 3- to 5-gallon (11–19 L) containers.

Plant ¼- to ½-inch (6–13 mm)-wide lateral roots cut into 6-inch (15 cm) segments. Bury the entire cutting at a 45-degree angle. The top should start about 2 inches (5 cm) under the soil.

In shallow soil, or when growing as a perennial, angled root corners or crowns can be planted. The top of the fat side should be about 2 inches (5 cm) deep. The lower side should be planted horizontally to encourage lateral, rather than vertical, growth.

Additionally, you can transplant young horseradish plants that sprout from the severed roots of a parent plant. Horseradish can be started from seed, too, though it may produce plants that are very different from their parent plants.

In hot areas, give plants full sun in cool weather. Then, provide partial shade when temperatures are over 80°F (27°C). Or grow from fall to spring in areas with no frosts.

To grow as a perennial, plants need 3–5 feet (91–152 cm) of space. In late fall, harvest the lateral roots located more than a 1-foot (30 cm) diameter away from the primary root as your harvest.

HARVESTING

Harvesting horseradish is all about root excavation. Act as if you are on an archaeological dig and carefully loosen and brush away soil to follow the full root length. If you leave any severed roots in the ground, they will eventually re-emerge as new plants.

Put fresh roots in a bucket of water to prevent the skins from drying. That way you can skip peeling them. Grate and preserve in vinegar.

You can store fresh horseradish in the fridge too. But its flavor and potency are stronger if it's preserved in vinegar immediately after harvesting.

MEDICINAL TIP

Horseradish's powerful stimulating effects make themselves known upon cutting into the pungent root. An antiviral herb that clears congestion and provokes secretion, it can aid in respiratory ailments when mucus is thick and obstructive.

You can make a traditional herbal preparation known as fire cider using freshly grated horseradish combined with spicy foods such as garlic, onion, hot peppers, and ginger, which is then steeped in vinegar. Temper it with a bit of honey. Then use as needed when a cold or flu hits.

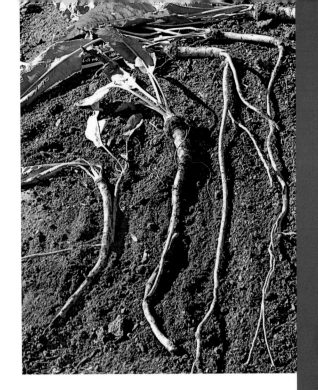

SPICE PROFILE
- **Name:** Horseradish
- **Latin:** *Armoracia rusticana* (syn. *Cochlearia armoracia*)
- **Native to:** southeastern Europe and Western Asia
- **Edible parts:** Entire plant
- **Culinary use:** Peppery, spicy, and slightly sweet with sinus-clearing attributes; used as a meat condiment

GROWING CONDITIONS
- Cool-season perennial, usually grown as an annual
- Mature plant tolerance -30–85°F (-1–29°C)
- Protect from prolonged heat
- Full sun to part shade; fertile, well-draining soil; pH 5.5–7.5
- 180+ days for large roots

ABOVE: *Horseradish roots grow impressively long. They can grow deep and laterally. The narrowest parts toward then ends can be cut into 6- to 8-inch (15–20 cm) pieces and used as seed stock for next year's plants.*

GARLIC— BEST ALL- PURPOSE SPICE

If I were stranded on a deserted island and could only have once spice, I'd choose garlic. And not just because I wouldn't have to worry about garlic breath! Garlic has excellent culinary diversity, medicinal value, and is easy to grow.

Also, contrary to popular belief, you can grow garlic in most climates with knowledge and the right seed stock. The four countries that garlic is native to have temperatures ranging from well below freezing to over 100° F (38°C). That gives you a sense of the conditions wild garlic can survive.

GARLIC TYPES

I could write a very long book on growing garlic, and, in fact, others have. For simplicity, though, garlic comes in two types: hardneck and softneck.

Softneck is most common because the cured heads store well. The soft green tops can be decoratively braided. However, in humid climates, braiding slows curing times and increases risk for rot.

In some growing conditions, softneck garlic will produce awkward, infertile bulbils midway up its green leaf stem. These will not grow new plants, but they are delicious too.

Hardneck garlic sends up flower stalks called scapes. These form flowers that open like fireworks (if not eaten first). The flowers give way to topsets. Topsets are tiny bulblets that form from the flowers. Some, though not all, hardneck garlic even produce small black seeds. Hardneck seeds and topsets can be planted. But it will take 2–3 years for a decent-sized head of garlic.

Hardnecks also make great perennials in temperate climates. If you leave the heads in the ground, each year new cloves will form.

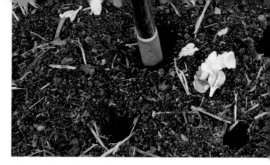

Use a rake end to poke holes to the right planting distance and depth in your prepared bed. Then, as you place a clove in each hole, cover it with soil to close the hole. When all your holes are covered with soil, water well. You can easily plant hundreds of cloves at a time this way.

Each clove will then send up a scape in spring. You can harvest all those scapes and cook them like asparagus to enjoy their mild garlic flavor.

For warm climates, opt for *creole* hardneck varieties. Store heads between 32–50° F (0–10°C) for 10–12 weeks before planting to vernalize. Otherwise, the plants will not bulb.

In moderate climates, with below freezing but overall mild winters, you can grow just about any garlic. However, you'll have the best luck with softnecks.

In cold climates, you can also grow most garlic types, though your bulb formation might not be as large as in moderate climates. Hardneck rocambole varieties will really shine.

GARLIC CARE

Garlic needs a long cool growing period. Plant it while days are short for good root development. Then, as days grow longer, bulbs will begin to form. Start garlic in early fall, about 4–6 weeks before first frost in cold areas. In frost-free areas, plant vernalized seed garlic during your coolest period starting in fall or early winter.

In very cold or hot climates, plant cloves 4 inches (10 cm) deep to protect from soil temperature fluctuations. In moderate climates, plant cloves 2 inches (5 cm) deep. Give each clove 4–5 inches (10–12.7 cm) of soil space between plants.

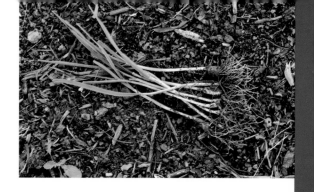

MEDICINAL TIP

Garlic and its medicinal powers have been revered throughout human history. In modern times, garlic supplementation has been popularized for its cardioprotective benefits, shown to decrease LDL cholesterol and triglyceride levels, while reducing inflammation and hypertension.[18] The antimicrobial properties of garlic, paired with its immune-boosting abilities, make this herb a top choice for fighting infections.[19] Consuming crushed raw garlic is the most potent way to eat this bulb, due to the allicin release that occurs.

SPICE PROFILE

- **Latin:** *Allium sativum*
- **Native to:** Kyrgyzstan, Tajikistan, Turkmenistan, and Uzbekistan
- **Edible parts:** Entire plant
- **Culinary use:** Tangy, peppery, spicy flavors become sweet and buttery when cooked; used for everything from savory dishes to ice cream

GROWING CONDITIONS

- Cool-season, day length dependent perennial, grown as an annual
- Mature plant tolerance -30–80°F (-1–27°C)
- Protect from excessive moisture and heat
- Full sun; fertile, well-draining soil; pH 6.0–7.5
- 180+ days for large heads

ABOVE: *Garlic plants are rarely started from seeds. Instead, we plant the individual cloves as "seed garlic." However, I did plant a patch of hardneck seeds for fun. A few germinated and produced these mild-tasting garlic plants.*

Water deeply to initiate root development. Then only water during extended drought.

About a month after planting, or just as the tips of the greens break ground, hoe your bed lightly to remove weeds. Then cover your bed with 2 inches (5 cm) of lightweight mulch such as straw or leaf compost between plants.

HARVESTING

Watch your garlic stems near the soil for signs of softening, bending, or slouching. Also watch leaves for yellowing at tips or streaking in their centers. Once this starts, harvest within a couple weeks, when the soil is dry and before big rains. For hardnecks, this happens shortly after the scapes emerge.

Loosen soil with a shovel or digging fork. Remove the entire garlic plant. Gently brush away the soil. Dry plants in the sun for a few hours. Then wipe each garlic head with a dry towel to remove dried dirt.

To cure garlic, hang garlic individually by its entire stem in a dry location out of direct light to cure. This takes about 2–3 weeks. Also, leave roots intact to act as a wick to draw moisture from the garlic heads.

Hardnecks have higher moisture content and are prone to rotting. Give them more room during drying. Hardnecks will store for 5–7 months. Softnecks can last for a year.

Trim roots and stems after curing. Store garlic in a cool, dry location. Save your largest, best garlic heads for planting. Then, at time of planting, open your heads and use only the largest cloves to start new plants.

LICORICE—
A NITROGEN-FIXING ROOT AND RHIZOME ALL-IN-ONE

Previously, I mentioned that licorice stores nutrients in its deep taproot. Amazingly, licorice (*Glycyrrhiza glabra*) also forms rhizomes that spread laterally to produce new plants. Commercial licorice growers often harvest only the rhizomes for sale to avoid disturbing the taproot.

This taproot/rhizome combo means licorice can potentially be even more invasive than horseradish in the right circumstances. However, licorice doesn't grow that easily except in its native Mediterranean-type habitat. Most of us will have to do a little work to grow licorice at home.

Seed Propagation

Stratify (cold treat) licorice seeds by putting them in a container of moist soil in the fridge for several weeks. Then rub seeds lightly

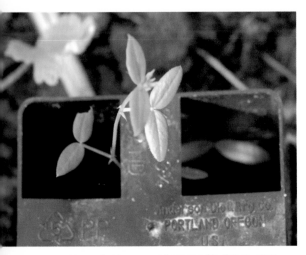

Young licorice grown from seed is slow to start and needs plenty of protection from weeds and harsh weather. Juvenile plants resemble other legumes such as peas and fenugreek. Young roots are carrotlike.

with sandpaper to *scarify* them. Finally, soak the seeds in warm water for several hours. Sow seeds ½ inch (12.7 mm) deep in loose soil. Water daily for several weeks until germination. Transplant to deeper pots before the roots outgrow the starter soil.

Vegetative Propagation

You can also start licorice from cuttings. Dormant 6- to 8-inch (15–20 cm) cuttings can go directly into the ground similar to the way horseradish is planted after risk of frost in spring. Smaller cuttings can be started in pots and transplanted once green tops and roots are established.

Planting beds or pots should be at least a foot deep, but preferably 2–3 feet (61–91 cm) deep for better root production. To harvest larger roots, space plants 1–2 feet (30–61 cm) apart. If you prefer to leave the root and harvest the rhizomes, then give plants 3–4 feet (91–122 cm) of space each.

In climates with winter lows above 15°, you can grow licorice in the ground year-round. For outdoor plant establishment, transplant or plant cuttings when temperatures will be between 40–80° (4–27°C) for at least 4 months to give young plants time to root.

In climates with cold winters, leave pots outside to vernalize when temperatures are above freezing. Bring pots in when temperatures are consistently below freezing. Return pots outdoors in warm weather.

Water regularly for the first 2 years. Then water only when the top few inches of soil are dry.

Note: Like fenugreek, licorice roots can coordinate with rhizobia bacteria to fix its own nitrogen. As such, in organic gardens use inoculant at planting and an annual dose of compost as fertilizer.

You can harvest the rhizomes and roots after 3 years. However, the medicinally potent glycyrrhizin will intensify if plants are grown for 5 years. Leave root portions or rhizomes in the soil so your licorice can self-renew. Or you can harvest everything and start again.

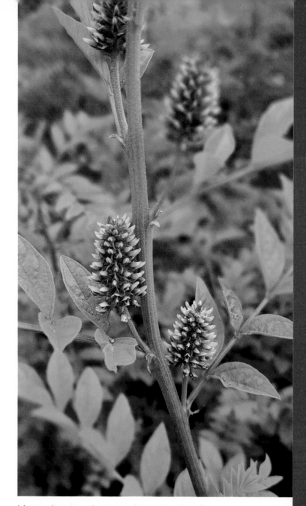

Mature licorice plants produce attractive flowers.

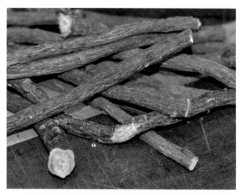

Mature licorice roots are long and narrow and can be cut into shorter segments for easier drying and storage.

MEDICINAL TIP

Licorice is a long-held staple in the herbal world, most commonly used for its demulcent activity, this plant shines in its ability to coat and soothe irritated tissue in the digestive and respiratory tracts. Use the dried root to make a sweet cup of tea. Use caution as high doses can cause pseudohyperaldosteronism, a condition that can lead to high blood pressure and other potentially serious side effects but that will cease once consumption is discontinued.

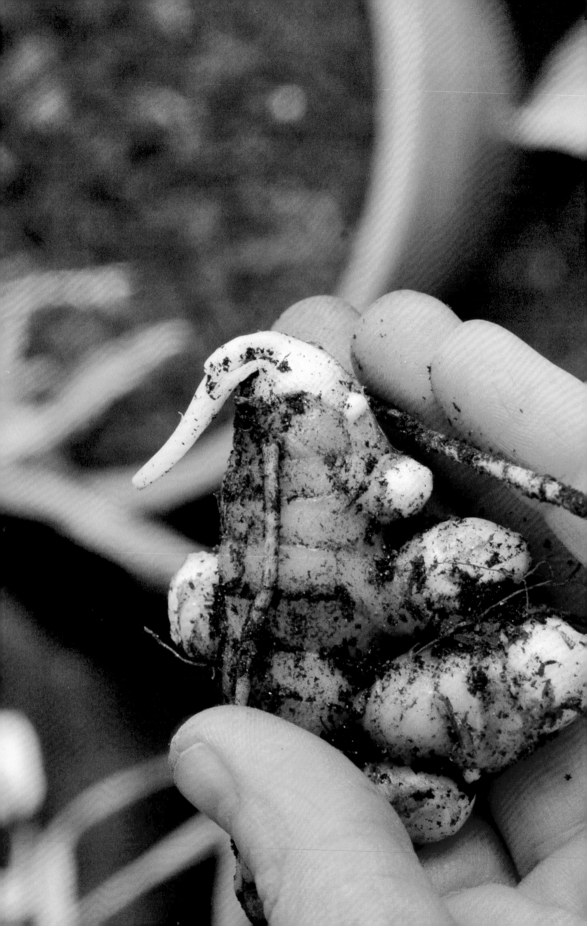

TROPICAL OR CONTAINER GROWN UNDERGROUND SPICES

These underground spices require warmer conditions to thrive. In temperate climates, you'll need to grow plants indoors part of the year to keep them alive.

< Turmeric "mothers" are as beautiful as they are productive.

GINGER— AN ANCIENT GMO

Ginger is native to nowhere. It's considered a *cultigen*, or a plant that exists as a result of human cultivation. We don't know its origin or when humans started using it. We only know that it would not exist without us.

Technically, cultigens have a lot in common with GMOs (genetically modified organisms). In both cases, human activity significantly alters the genetic make-up of a plant species to the point that it becomes an entirely new plant.

The primary distinction, though, is that with cultigens, we don't know when or where those plants crossed into "new" territory. Related plants were likely cultivated for thousands of generations before that magical moment. Only in deep time does a plant like ginger becomes so distinguished from its near relatives that we consider it a human creation.

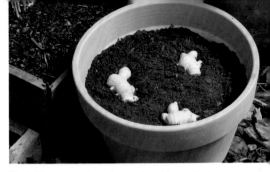

Start rhizomes indoors in a pot and transplant outdoors in warm weather. Select fat rhizome pieces with multiple eyes. Fill pot with soil to 2 inches (5 cm) from the top. Apply slow-release fertilizer and set the rhizome cuttings on the fertilized soil. Top pot with compost.

With GMOs, by contrast, new plants are made in laboratories in a single generation. Often the genetic alterations are so well documented, or even marked with a DNA signature, that we can identify them anywhere they grow. Still, there may come a time when GMOs are so common that we do lose track of them. Then, future humans might call our modern-day GMOs cultigens.

GINGER CARE

Even though ginger is a cultigen, there are also many *cultivars* of ginger. Cultivars are plants that have been cultivated for specific qualities such a taste, color, and storage qualities. The ginger in most grocery stores are Chinese types. These are mild tasting and have thick skins for longer shelf-life.

Any market ginger can be planted if it is not diseased or old. However, mature rhizomes that have been through natural *senescence* will produce the best yields. Senescence typically happens in fall after plants have had a long growing season. Waning daylight and cooling soil temperatures signal ginger to prepare rhizomes to survive until optimal conditions come again.

During senescence, leaves will begin to yellow and brown as their energy is redirected to the rhizomes. That's when rhizomes develop their protective skins. This is also when seed ginger is harvested.

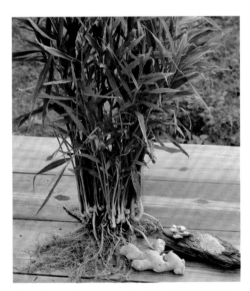

Ginger is used fresh, cured, dried, and powdered. The rhizomes can be eaten young or after senescence. You can even eat the shoots (which are really leaves, called *psuedostems*) chopped.

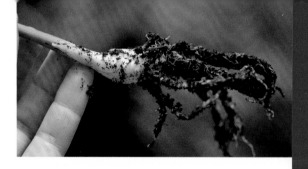

MEDICINAL TIP

Ginger, while well known for its use in allaying nausea and vomiting, is also renowned for its impressive virucidal properties.[20] The most effective way to receive this medicine is through the use of its fresh juice. Process the root with a juicer, place the liquid in ice cube trays, and store in the freezer to have an easily accessible antiviral remedy on hand. Add water, honey, and a squeeze of lemon to cut the spiciness as needed.

SPICE PROFILE
- **Names:** Ginger Root, Ginger Rhizome
- **Latin:** *Zingiber officinale*
- **Native to:** Non-native cultigen
- **Edible parts:** Entire plant
- **Culinary use:** Spicy, sweet, and tangy taste is used for curries, cookies, salad dressings, beverages, and more

GROWING CONDITIONS
- Subtropical/Tropical perennial, grown as an annual
- Mature plant tolerance 35–105°F (2–41°C); needs temperatures above 65 °F (18°C) for growth
- Part shade to full sun; fertile, well-draining soil; pH 5.5–6.5
- Start from rhizome cuttings; 200+ days to harvest

Ginger can survive almost to freezing if there is no frost. However, it only grows well in temperatures above 65° (18°C).

To start in midwinter, obtain post-senescence-harvested rhizomes. Store them in a warm, indirectly lit location until the eyes develop. For grocery store ginger, soak for 24 hours, replacing the water every few hours, to expunge growth retardants. Cut or break rhizomes into 2-ounce (56.7 g) pieces that contain 1–3 eyes. Allow the cuts 1–2 days to crust.

ABOVE: *Young ginger produces underground nodes. Each individual node can be separated and transplanted to form a new ginger plant. However, starting plants from 2 ounce (56.7 g) cuttings will provide a bigger harvest.*

Plant your rhizome cuttings 1–2 inches (2.5–5 cm) deep in prepared beds or containers. Keep the soil uniformly moist until shoots emerge in about a month. Ginger can grow 2–5 (61–91 cm) feet tall.

When growing in the ground, periodically hill the soil from the outer edges of your rows around the root area to encourage the rhizomes to plump. Stop fertilizing if plants flower.

HARVESTING
Baby ginger can be harvested in 6–8 months. Dig and harvest rhizome pieces pre-senescence for fresh use.

Mature ginger takes 10-plus months. Dig up entire rhizome and roots after senescence. Save your fattest, healthiest rhizomes as seed stock.

To initiate premature senescence, cut the top few inches of leaves to reduce photosynthesis. Then harvest in 2–3 weeks.

TURMERIC— A DELIGHT TO THE HEART

According to researchers, turmeric has at least 53 different names in Sanskrit.[i] Many of the translations are descriptive such as *gives the golden color, greenish, reddish brown*, and *long in appearance*. Others relate to its utility such as *which cures fevers, clears darkness and imparts color, killer of fat*, and *killer of worms*.

My favorite Sanskrit translations, though, are the personal and poetic descriptors such as *as beautiful as moonlight, dear to hari, Lord Krishna, gives delight to the heart*, and *beloved of wife*. These terms convey the deeply important role turmeric has held in Hindu culture.

Turmeric is so much more than a spice. It's used as a coloring agent, in religious celebrations, as a healing medicine, and in beauty products. It stains the hands of those who harvest and process it marking them as the caretakers of this golden cultigen.

TURMERIC CARE

Turmeric and ginger require the same growing cultures. Rather than reiterate that information, please refer to the ginger profile for care details before starting turmeric. However, there are a few important differences from ginger that earn turmeric its own profile.

SEED TURMERIC

Unlike ginger, which can be grown from any part of a post-senescent rhizome, starting turmeric from a mother is better. The mother is the central body from which the fingers, or baby rhizomes, of turmeric grow. The mother gets more productive each year that it is grown.

Turmeric fingers can also be planted. However, fingers still need to mature into mothers before they begin their reproductive process. This means the fingers will be later

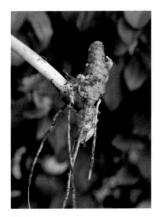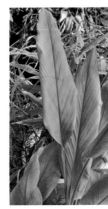

LEFT: This plant was started from a turmeric finger. It's small in size and will be slow to start producing fingers. Each year it will become more productive as it matures. Save your mature mothers to replant each year.

RIGHT: Senescence is easy to see on turmeric leaves. As the chlorophyll wanes, the leaves begin to lighten and brown at the edges.

to start and smaller in size than those produced by a mature mother.

Start growing mothers in mid- to late winter. Start growing fingers at the beginning of winter to give them more time to mature. Then, care for turmeric like ginger.

PLANTING MARKET TURMERIC

You can plant fresh turmeric from the market, but you'll want to buy it early in winter. If you try to plant market turmeric that you find in midsummer, it will likely go dormant before producing many (or any) fingers. You'd have to grow it again the following year to achieve good yields.

HARVESTING TURMERIC

Turmeric is only harvested post-senescence (after the leaves die back). In most climates this happens in fall. However, there are some early varieties that will develop fingers by summer.

You'll know when to harvest turmeric by the leaves. When they begin to yellow throughout and brown at the edges, harvesting can begin. Use your hands to dig the rhizomes out of the loose soil you planted them in.

Keep your mothers for replanting in winter. Use turmeric fingers for grating fresh into dishes or making into a powder. Store fresh turmeric in your crisper drawer in the fridge.

POWDERING TURMERIC

Fresh turmeric must be boiled and then dried to make powdered turmeric. First, barely cover the fingers with water. Boil over low heat, and continue to boil only until the rhizomes are tender and begin to release a fragrant aroma. Overcooking diminishes the flavor and fragrance.

Once cooked, allow turmeric to dry in a dark location at about 60°F (16°C). Warmer drying temperatures are said to weaken the flavor. You can use a fan on a low setting to shorten drying time. Depending on your conditions, drying can take 5–15 days.

After drying, grind the fingers into powder using your spice grinder or a mortar and pestle.

MEDICINAL TIP

A traditional and long-standing medicine in Ayurveda, turmeric is one of the top-selling herbal supplements in America.[21] It's endorsed in the West for its efficacy at reducing joint pain in inflammatory conditions such as arthritis.[22] The antioxidant activity can also help stave off degenerative illnesses associated with aging.[23] Its established use in cream-laden Indian dishes is a great extraction method for the fat-soluble compounds of turmeric; add in a dash of black pepper to increase absorption.

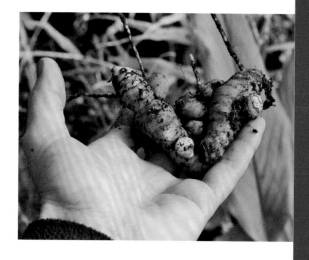

SPICE PROFILE
- **Names:** Turmeric root, Curcumin, Indian Saffron
- **Latin:** *Curcuma longa*
- **Native to:** Non-native cultigen
- **Edible parts:** Entire plant
- **Culinary use:** Smokey, mouth-drying, pungent; used for curries, coloring, rice dishes, and as a daily medicinal supplement

GROWING CONDITIONS
- Subtropical/Tropical perennial, grown as an annual
- Mature plant tolerance 35–105°F (2–41°C); needs temperatures above 65 °F (18°C) for growth
- Part shade to full sun; fertile, well-draining soil; pH 5.5–6.5
- Start from mothers or fingers; 200+ days to harvest

ABOVE: *The central body of this rhizome is a turmeric mother. The fingers grow from her sides. In my greenhouse, the fingers fatten first on the south-facing side, then fill in on the north side. This growth habit always makes me think of a litter of piglets nursing from their mother.*

CARDAMOM— CULTURAL EYE OPENER

I spent a college semester in Washington, D.C., sharing an apartment with a Catholic from Kentucky, a Jew from New Jersey, and a Muslim from Morocco, and I was a "Questioning" from California. It sounds like the start of a bad joke. But that experience taught me that *variety is the spice of life.*

For my Moroccan roommate's birthday, her visiting mother and aunt occupied our kitchen to make a feast of varied vegetables, meats, fish, and sweets. When their efforts were revealed, every dish was an exploration in spice. I still fantasize about the cardamom-spiced dishes I sampled that night.

Later, while living in Egypt, I ate similar dishes made by an Algerian chef. After that, I assumed that cardamom was a North African-grown spice. While researching this book, I discovered that Guatemala, a country whose people use very little cardamom, is the largest producer. Large quantities of cardamom are also grown in India, though most of it is consumed locally.

When I think of cardamom's native range of Ceylon and India, the heavy use in Arab culture, global export production in Guatemala, and my experiences eating it in Washington, D.C., and Egypt, these famous lyrics ring true: *It's a small world after all.*

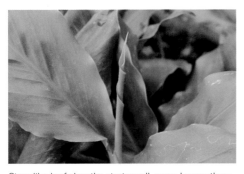

Strawlike leaf sheaths start small, grow larger, then open like flowers.

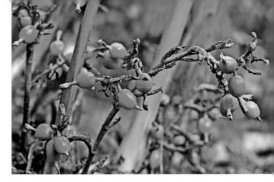

Cardamom flowers and pods are produced low on the plant. The pods should be harvested before they split.

Cardamom, the plant, however, is not. It can range from 6–16 feet (1.8–5 m) tall before it puts out pods. Plan to give it plenty of space!

CARDAMOM CARE

Cardamom grows like ginger. However, it is not a cultigen, as wild populations of cardamom still exist. Additionally, since we harvest the pods, the flowers require insect or hand-pollination to produce pods.

Cultivated cardamom stays beautiful year-round if kept above 50°F (10°C). That makes it a great choice as a space filling tropical plant indoors and out. It also requires part shade and can be grown near a sunny window without supplemental electric light.

Cardamom grows tall, not by elongating stems, but by layered leaf sheaths. Essentially, a series of leaves rolled up like overlapping straws shoot up from the rhizome. Underground rhizomes move laterally in the soil, sending up new leaf sheaths.

In ideal conditions, plants flower in year 2 or 3 and reach full production in year 4. They continue to produce for 10–15 years. Flowers arch out from the base like spider legs. In less than ideal conditions, fruiting may be irregular.

You can start cardamom by seed. Lightly scarify seeds and then sow in 70–80°F (21–27°C) soil, ¼ inch (6 mm) deep. Keep soil moist until germination (20–45 days). Germination rates are low, so plant extras.

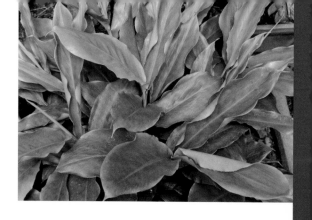

New plants can also be made by dividing old plants. Loosen the soil around the parent plant. Separate a rhizome segment with 4–5 leaf sheaths and establish that in a new location.

To grow cardamom indoors, use a wide, relatively deep container to retain moisture and accommodate its mature size. Plants also need vertical space in their third year and beyond.

These plants are surface feeders. Use compost tea weekly and top off pots with organic matter (compost, leaf mulch, or light wood mulch) to keep the soil level. Water regularly.

HARVESTING

Flowering begins in early spring through summer. Then it takes 120-plus days for the pods to mature. Harvest when the seeds inside are dark brown to black and before the pods split. Mature pods are easy to hand-pick; immature pods hang on tight.

At home, winnow your pods and rinse them quickly in cold water. Dry them on a baking sheet in your oven or in your dehydrator at temperatures of 90–125°F (32–52°C).

SPICE PROFILE
- **Names:** Green, White, or True Cardamom
- **Latin:** *Elettaria cardamomum*
- **Native to:** South India and Ceylon
- **Edible parts:** Pods, seeds, possibly roots, and leaves
- **Culinary use:** Sweet, floral, lemony with a hint of mint and black pepper, used for desserts, meats, and in coffee

GROWING CONDITIONS
- Subtropical/Tropical perennial
- Mature plant tolerance 40–95°F (4–35°C); 60–85°F (16–29°C) required for growth
- 40–60% shade; fertile, well-draining soil; pH 4.5–6.5
- Start from plant divisions or seeds; 3+ years to harvest

ABOVE: *Cardamom is a lovely plant even when it's not flowering. Its mounding habit and lush leaves add interest to a tropical container garden or greenhouse.*

MEDICINAL TIP

Cardamom can be used as a mouthwash or part of a tooth powder recipe to invoke its antimicrobial properties in tooth infections all the while strengthening gums and freshening breath.[24] The aromatic oils of cardamom are also beneficial in cases of atonic dyspepsia (indigestion), with stomach pains and flatulence.[25] Add a pinch of ground cardamom to your warm beverages for its pungent flavor and medicinal benefits or utilize capsules for larger doses.

Pods have about 85 percent moisture to start and should end up at about 10–12 percent moisture. Weigh your batch of pods before and after drying to confirm moisture content.

If you decorticate, or hull your pods, seeds lose volatile oils quickly. Instead keep the pods intact until needed.

WASABI FOR EVERYONE!

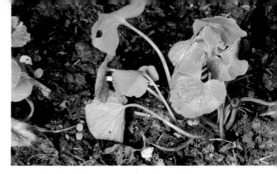

Wasabi plantlets need time to establish deep roots before the fattened wasabi stem forms. In dry areas, install a drip line at the root zone and water all of the soil regularly for faster growth rates.

Saffron is the most expensive spice in the world in terms of weight. Wasabi, however, is the rarest in terms of production. Most of what is labeled as *wasabi* is a combination of horseradish, mustard, and food coloring.

Real wasabi is primarily cultivated in its native homeland of Japan. Due to culinary popularity, countries such as the U.S., New Zealand, China, Vietnam, Israel, Canada, and Australia have also dabbled in growing wasabi.

Generally, most people believe wasabi production is limited because of the difficulty of growing this semi-aquatic plant outside Japan. However, the truth is, it's not difficult to grow wasabi if you know how.

Young wasabi plants start settling in by forming deep roots in loose soil. Then leaves begin to grow. In a few months, a stubby stalk becomes obvious above the soil line. As older leaves grow large, age, and die, newer leaves form from the top center of the aboveground stem.

Slowly, the stubby stalk gets incrementally taller. When the dead, withered leaves fall away, ridges or scales remains on the stalk. The aboveground stalk is actually a fattened stem, often referred to as a rhizome, that we think of as wasabi. This leaf-molting/stalk-growing process gives mature wasabi the appearance of a miniature palm tree with rounded leaves.

WASABI CARE

To start wasabi at home, find a seller of the plantlets. Unless you can pick them up locally, plantlets are usually shipped in cool temperatures.

You will need to grow wasabi mostly outdoors, in a shaded area such as under an outcropping of trees. You will also need to water often. So, easy access to cold water is important.

You can plant well-rooted wasabi plantlets in the ground, in raised beds, or in containers. Containers are necessary in cold climates as you'll need to bring plants indoors if temperatures drop below 30° F (-1°C). Indoors, place plants next to a window on the shady side of your home.

Wasabi likes good garden soil that is heavily amended with leaf mulch, peat moss, or perlite to improve drainage. Make sure you can pour a gallon or two of water through your soil mix without it becoming boggy before planting.

Plant the wasabi root line slightly above the soil level. It will settle a bit when you water. Do not cover any part of the above ground stem or this might cause rotting. Mulch with small pebbles to preserve moisture. This also protects the above-ground wasabi stem from sinking when watered.

Water wasabi daily with cold water to keep the roots and soil cool. Water twice daily, with cold water, on hot days. Use compost tea or other liquid fertilizers weekly to replace nutrients lost to frequent watering.

STARTING WASABI FROM SEED

To start wasabi from seed, place 15–20 seeds in a 4-inch (10 cm) container of prepared soil. Cover seeds with a sprinkle of compost and a layer of chicken grit to protect it during heavy watering.

Place pots in a shady location outdoors in late winter or early spring to vernalize. Water enough to keep the soil moist until seeds sprout; this generally takes several months. When seedlings have established roots, treat them like plantlets.

HARVESTING

Harvest your fresh wasabi in 1½–3 years, depending on desired size. Harvest the entire plant. Snap off your best plantlets and start replacement plants.

Trim the leaves and roots. Before grating, use a sharp knife to scrape off the ridged leaf nodes on the stem. Use a wasabi grater or cheese grater to shred your wasabi.

According to Japanese tradition, you must grate wasabi with a smile. Also, inhale deeply as you do to clear your sinus passages. Eat within 15 minutes of grating. Wrap unused portions in wet newspaper and store in your crisper for up to 2 weeks.

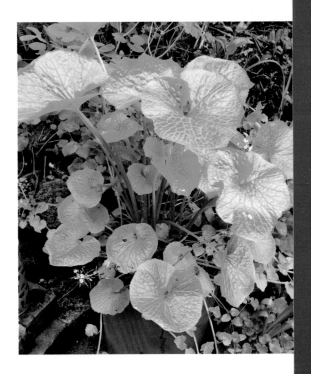

SPICE PROFILE
- **Names:** Japanese horseradish
- **Latin:** *Eutrema japonicum* (syn. *Wasabia japonica*)
- **Native to:** Japan
- **Edible parts:** Entire plant
- **Culinary use:** Spicy, burning, hot mustard taste used for sushi

GROWING CONDITIONS
- Subtropical perennial
- Mature plant tolerance 27–80° (-3–27°C); ideal range 45–65° (7–18°C)
- Full shade; fertile, moist soil; pH 6.0–7.0
- Start from plantlets or seeds; 18+ months to harvest

ABOVE: *Wasabi plants can be grown in containers or in the ground. This plant will soon be ready to harvest.*

MEDICINAL TIP

Wasabi, while elusive outside of its native region, has established uses in herbal medicine. Highlighted for its rich poly-phenol content,[26] wasabi effectively scavenges free radicals verifying its traditional uses of increasing longevity and health in those who consume it. Its anti-inflammatory activity is highly active throughout the nervous system and works to reduce neuroinflammation in the brain.[27] Use homegrown wasabi grated fresh whenever a harvest is possible.

GROW YOUR OWN
TOM KHA GAI THEMED SPICE GARDEN

If you love Tom Kha Gai (coconut Thai soup), those signature flavors are perfect for a themed spice garden. The main flavoring agents—galangal, Thai bird chilis, cilantro, kaffir lime leaves, and lemon grass—are also useful in a host of other Asian-inspired dishes and are easy to grow.

Kaffir lime likes semi-dry Mediterranean conditions, similar to bay laurel (see the next section) when grown in the ground. But if it's container-grown, it needs a deep pot, applications of citrus fertilizer during leafing and fruiting, and consistent watering.

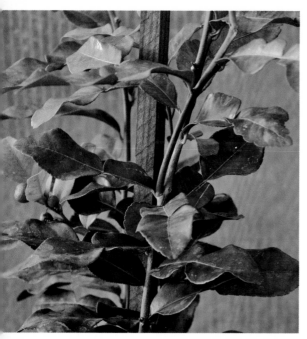

The thick, double-lobed evergreen leaves of this kaffir lime citrus tree is the primary spice. The rinds of the fruit are also fragrant and tasty, though not as commonly used.

Refer to the coriander and paprika profiles to grow your cilantro and bird chilis. Since coriander is a cool-season plant, grow it in the part shade of the kaffir lime and water it regularly to prevent bolting. Harvest the young leaves and replant often for a continuous supply.

Lemongrass, typically grown from seed for its aboveground, aromatic stalks, likes the same growing conditions as ginger. Just give it full sun for best results.

Growing Galangal

Galangal (*Alpinia galangal*) is grown from rhizome cuttings in conditions just like ginger. However, you'll grow it as a perennial. Allow it to establish in a large pot or deep bed for at least a year before you begin harvesting.

Unlike ginger, don't harvest post-senescence. Rhizomes that harden in response to cooler conditions are difficult to cut. Instead, harvest the new, tender rhizome growth from the second year on.

Galangal can't overwinter in frozen soil. But it can go dormant and survive temperatures as low as 25°F (-4°C). For ideal growth, keep it in the 50–85° F (10–29°C) range. Like cardamom, this plant prefers part shade or filtered light over direct sun.

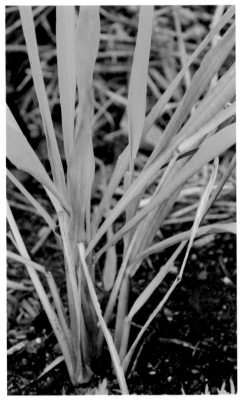

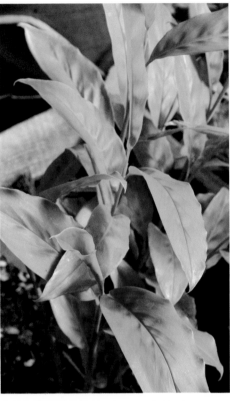

Lemongrass looks much like other clumping grasses. It grows quickly in heat and is not frost-hardy. Unlike other grasses, though, its fragrant stems are unmistakably lemon-scented and spicy-sweet tasting.

Galangal is not quite as showy as its cardamom cousin. But it also puts on a lovely leaf display during the growing season.

Harvesting Galangal

Gently dig around the rhizome mass to break off small pieces when you need them. Replace the soil and wait a day or two before watering to allow the exposed rhizome edge to harden. Give the plant time to recover before harvesting again. Slice and dry extra galangal harvested. Rehydrate prior to use.

Other Galangals

Other unique tasting galangals such as *Kaempferia galangal*, *Alpinia officinarum*, and *Boesenbergia rotunda* can be grown similarly.

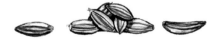

SECTION 3
PERENNIAL SPICES

Growing a perennial plant, particularly one not adapted to your climate, is much like pre-industrial spice exploration. You'll spend several years of your life in pursuit of something that may or may not bear the fruit you expect.

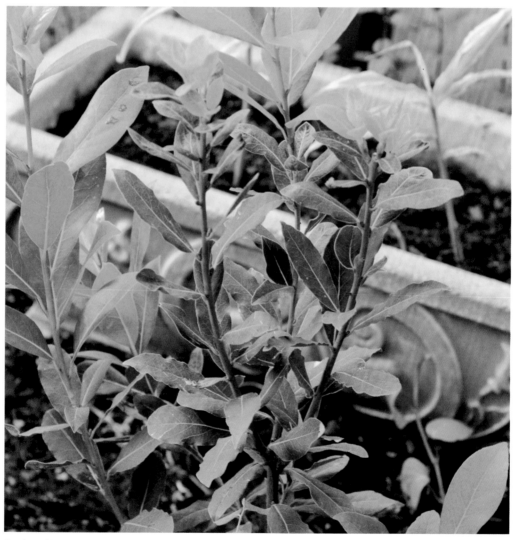

Bay laurel is an easy-care perennial that can grow into a large shrub or tree in frost-free regions.

Take Christopher Columbus, for example. He and a crew set sail to find a shorter route to transport black pepper from Malabar to Europe. Instead, they discovered a route to the Americas. That event led to the introduction of things such as chocolate, chili peppers, and vanilla to the global spice trade.

Growing exotic perennial spices is not as risky as a long sea voyage using only a compass, star navigation skills, and your dreams of glory to guide you. And you aren't as likely to become a controversial historic figure whose legacy is still revered and reviled today.

You will risk an investment of resources such as your valuable time without any assurances of success. It's also a labor of love. You may spend more to grow some spices in this section in than it costs you to buy them. Plus, you're likely to suffer a few setbacks until you better understand each plant's needs.

This isn't meant as discouragement. Growing these spices has been a source of joy and endless fascination for me, and I believe they will be for you too. Inherent challenges aside, committing to long-term relationship with your plants is one of the easiest ways to truly test your gardening mettle. Also, as with any good journey, the experience is often more rewarding than reaching your destination.

Start your adventure knowing that the real benefit of growing perennial spices is the lessons they will teach you about how to (and sometimes how *not* to) be a better gardener.

TECHNIQUES FOR GROWING PERENNIAL SPICES

If you are ready to grow your skills as a gardener, then let's start our perennial spice journey with a look at those inherent challenges I mentioned.

PLANT AVAILABILITY

Many perennial spices are still grown in semi-wild conditions. Growers may propagate new plants from their best-producing specimens, but they aren't intensively breeding plants the way growers do staples such as corn and soybeans or beloved hydrangeas and roses. That means these plants may not have a great deal of genetic diversity and tend to be adapted for very specific climates. Plants may also be hard to find given the limited number of growers.

For best results, ask sellers for details about the soil medium, fertilization, watering needs, light conditions, and temperatures in which those plants have been raised. Then aim to match those conditions at home.

PROPAGATION

Propagating perennial spices also requires special techniques. Even if you buy plants, understanding propagation techniques can help you tailor your care approach.

Seed Starting

Seed-grown plants may be hardier and somewhat adaptable to different environments than clones. Unfortunately, seed-grown plants that are heterozygous (carry the genetic coding from both parent plants) may take traits from each parent plant. As such, the productivity, flavor profile, and even the sex of some plants won't be known until they flower and fruit.

You can care for perennial seedlings as you would annual seed spices. But you may need to use special germination procedures and wait longer for germination. Here are some seed-starting methods you may need.

- Scarification is a process of wearing away the seed shell to help water penetrate and trigger germination. Use fine sandpaper to gently remove part of the protective outer seed layer.

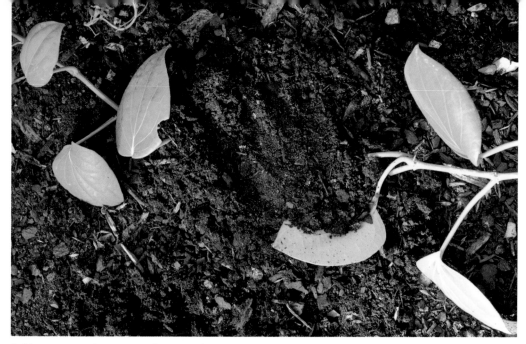

Soil layering new plants is easy. Remove a few leaves and press the bare node area into soil. Cover the soil with a weight if necessary. Leave the node in place until roots form. Vines such as black pepper (shown) or vanilla are easy to practice this technique with since they have aerial roots already.

• Soaking pre-treatment softens the seed shell.

• Sellers may recommend hot water soaking. While this may kill bacterial or fungal pathogens, unfortunately, it can also reduce germination rates. Start extra seeds as precaution.

• Stratification is like vernalization for seeds. The most common method is to put seeds in a container of damp planting medium and store in the fridge. This simulates overwintering in winter soil. You can also stratify seeds outdoors in winter.

• Like other spices grown from seed. specific amounts of light and the right soil temperatures are still required to germinate.

Layering

Layering is a method of propagation done using the stems or branches of a living plant while they are still attached to the plant.

This form of asexual reproduction produces a clone of the parent.

Layering takes from 3–24 months depending on the plant. Production is also limited to layering a few branches at a time to avoid harming the parent plant.

Soil Layering

To layer in the ground soil or in a pot, fold a pliable, young but not new growth area of the stem to the soil level. Remove a few leaves from a middle section of the stem and push the leafless nodes into the medium. Use a rock or other weight to hold the nodes in the soil.

Changing the stem angle and allowing nodes to be in contact with soil triggers the plant to make roots rather than new leaves. Once the stem has roots, cut it away from the parent plant and grow it as a separate plant.

Air Layering

To air layer, remove a section of the outer bark from a branch and scrape away the green cambium layer underneath. This girdles that section of the tree to slow its nutrient flow. Then wrap the barkless section with moist planting medium fastened in place with plastic or aluminum wrap. Once roots form from the girdled area, cut below the roots and pot your new tree.

For post-layering care, keep new plants in the same growing conditions as the parent plant. Note: layered plants generally carry the same diseases as the parent. Use only healthy, disease-free plants for layering.

Cuttings

Propagating by cuttings is a variation on layering. The difference is you use sections of freshly cut stems to regrow plants. See the lavender profile for full details.

Tissue Cloning

Tissue cloning is done in a petri dish. A small portion of a plant is used to isolate cells that are then added to a nutritive growing medium. The cells grow and divide until they eventually make new plants. Once the cells form a plant, the clones are potted and grown in nurseries.

The benefit of tissue cloning is that cells can be taken from disease-free segments of the cloned parent plant, thereby reducing pathogen risks. Also, thousands of plants can be made from small sections of a single parent plant.

The challenge with tissue-cloned plants is that they are grown in highly regulated conditions. They are also typically sold as small plants since they take so long to grow. As such, grow tissue clones in protected conditions until they size up. Then harden them off before exposing them to direct sunlight or variable weather conditions.

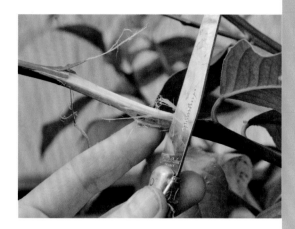

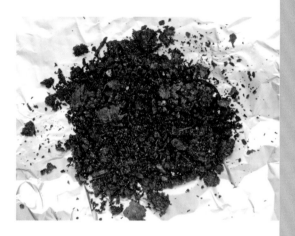

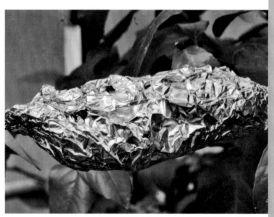

You can air layer sturdy stems by removing the bark and cambium of a branch and wrapping moist rooting medium over the wound until roots form.

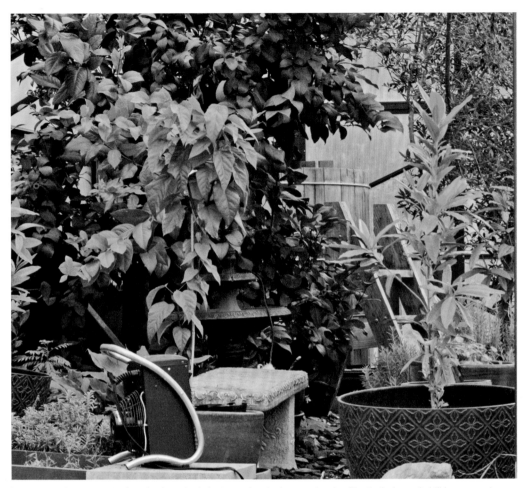

In my greenhouse, tropical and subtropical plants are located near a heater. Plants that need chill hours are in unheated zones. Water drums, a fountain, a hot tub, and active compost piles increase humidity and regulate temperatures. A mix of large pots and in-ground plants foster various hot, cool, dry, and moist conditions.

CLIMATE CONDITIONS

Perennial spice plants require specific climate conditions year-round. Here are the basic conditions for each climate type.

Tropical

Tropical plants require average temperatures above 64°F (18°C) even in winter. Temperatures between 75–85° F (24–29°C) are ideal for growth. Relative humidity above 60 percent and regular watering is required.

Subtropical

Subtropical plants can tolerate temperatures down to 32°F (0°C) but need consistent winter temperatures between 55–65°F (13–18°C). Temperatures between 70–85°F (21–29°C) are ideal for growth. Relative humidity above 60 percent is preferable. Water regularly.

Mediterranean

Mature Mediterranean plants can tolerate temperatures down to 25°F (-4°C), with average cold season temperatures around 45°F (7°C) .

Temperatures of 65–80°F (18–27°C) and relative humidity close to 60% are ideal for growth. Consistent watering is beneficial as plants are putting on new leaves. Otherwise only water when the soil begins to dry at the surface.

Temperate
Temperate climates have below freezing winters and warm to hot summers. Temperate plant requirements can vary widely. These plants may require vernalization, also called chill hours in perennial fruiting plants, to trigger new leaf and flower production. Chill hours are calculated as the number of hours when temperatures range between 32–45°F (0–7°C) in winter. Check with plant and seed sellers to find out the number of chill hours required before purchase to make sure you can provide those conditions at home.

MATURE PLANT SIZE
Some perennial spice plants can grow to 30 feet (9.1 m) or taller in the ground. However, often they can be kept small by growing them in tree-sized containers and pruning regularly. For meaningful production, grow trees to at least 5–8 (1.5–2.4 m) feet tall.

PRUNING
Perennial spice trees and shrubs require regular pruning. I recommend new gardeners find a good pruning guide to help you get started. I've posted some pruning guides on my website www.simplestead.com. Also, agricultural universities and forestry services often have useful pruning guides.

In the meantime, here are some tips to get you started. Additional tips are included on some of the profiles.

• Review the sanitation section in "Basic Spice Care."

• To control for size, prune when the plant is dormant. Or prune immediately after flowering.

• To encourage bushiness, prune growing tips when a plant is actively growing.

• Avoid major pruning in late summer or fall when plants need their leaves to photosynthesize stored sugars in preparation for a winter rest.

• Prune damaged leaves or branches anytime to prevent pathogen transmission.

WINTER CARE
All plants have a slow period when they grow less. Even evergreens will look a little lackluster and drop some leaves. This is usually in the winter.

During this natural downtime, avoid fertilizing. Only water when the soil dries in the top 1–2 inches (2.5–5 cm). When your plant starts forming new leaf buds, begin fertilizing and watering normally again.

EXPEDITED SPICE PRODUCTION
If you are eager for production, buy the most mature plants you can find. It's tempting to buy a $10 seedling or a pack of seeds rather than spend $100 for a ready-to-produce plant. However, when you value the time and care you'll spend to grow a perennial spice to maturity, those seemingly expensive larger plants are almost always a bargain.

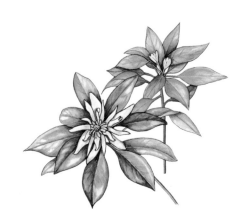

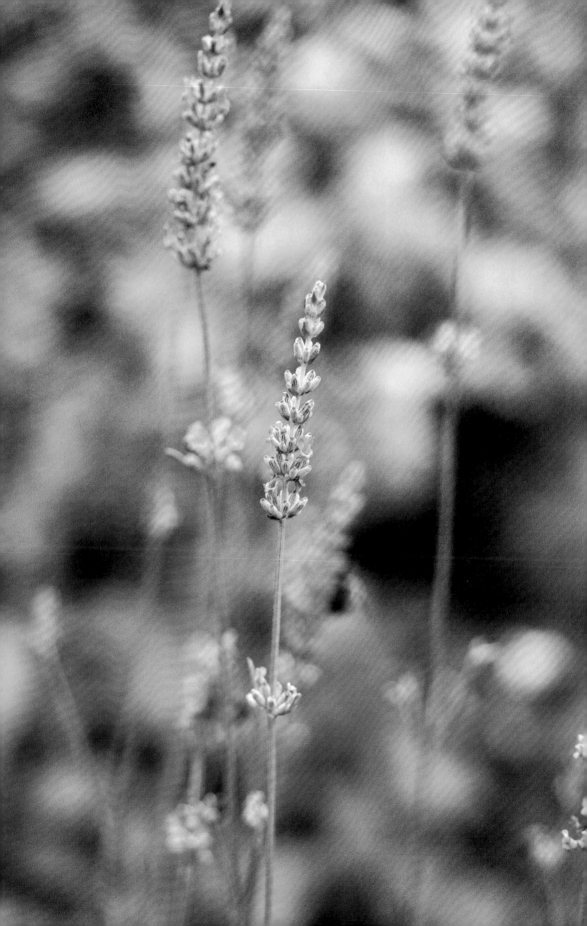

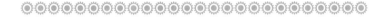

MEDITERRANEAN AND TEMPERATE CLIMATE PERENNIAL SPICES

The spice plants in this section have some cold tolerance. Some may also require winter chill hours for leaf set, flowering, and fruit production.

< Lavender wands are ready to harvest when one or two flower buds open and the rest are plump. Dry the wand, then remove the buds to use as spice.

CAPERS—
UNDER THE
TUSCAN SUN

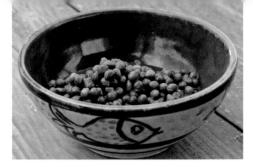

Caper buds come in many sizes. For peak tenderness, the smaller buds are better. Pickle or salt-pack to preserve them.

Enormous caper plants grow in bits of soil found in rock crevices along salty coast lines. A seed finds its way into that perfect spot and then spends several years biding its time until the conditions are perfect for germination. On a mildly warm day, a pleasant Mediterranean late winter rain finally penetrates the weathered seed shell. The once-dormant seed is spurred to action by an enzymatic reaction that triggers the cycle of growth.

If you were to take this same seed and start it in plenty of potting soil and give it all the care as you would cumin, you will likely fail. Capers are born to be wild. Respect their rugged individuality and mimic their natural preferences by using seed scarification and soaking. Then plant those seeds in rocky sparse soils, to get them started.

I also believe capers crave the beauty and simplicity of rustic living. That's why they grow like weeds in ancient villages under the Tuscan sun. So you'll also want to create a Tuscan environment for them to thrive. Caper plants can be tricky to start, yet with clever care, you can enjoy this nonpareil (unparalleled) taste of Tuscany no matter where you live.

CAPER CARE

Capers are xerophytic meaning adapted to grow with very little water. They are perfect for growing in a xeriscape (a landscape full of dry-loving plants) or a rock garden. Unfortunately, capers are not cold hardy and require Mediterranean winters to thrive. Capers also don't love humidity.

Thankfully, capers can be grown in pots so you can better control environmental conditions. For your first season, protect your caper plants from harsh winds and water deeply every week or two while they are putting on new leaves. After that, water only when the top 2 inches (5 cm) of soil are dry.

Keep mature plants in full sun in a breezy area to reduce humidity. Protect capers by moving them under cover on rainy days. Or make yourself a polycarbonate pergola under which you can grow all your Mediterranean plants.

My capers grow best in a mix of aged compost and gravel or potting mix with compost and gravel. Warning! Roly polies (*Armadillilium vulgare*) love tasty caper leaves. Because these (mostly) beneficial garden helpers require moist areas to thrive, surround the crown of the plant with large rocks that heat up dry quickly in sun. Capers also love to grow in deep, wide terracotta pots.

Don't lose hope if your capers seem nearly dormant at first. These plants focus on root development over leaf development as a survival strategy. They may only put on a few leaves for months, then in their second and third year, leaf mass will be more abundant.

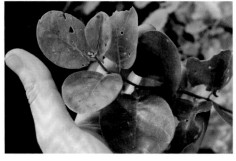

Caper leaves are tasty treats for us and for leaf-eating insects and birds. You may need to protect young caper plants from pests until they have abundant leaf growth.

HARVESTING CAPERS

For the pickled capers you find in stores, the fattened but not-yet-opened flower buds are harvested. These are graded, with the smallest unopened buds being the best. These are called nonpareil and are under ¼ inch (6 mm) in size. They are followed in size-order grading by surfines, capucines, capotes, fines, and grusas. Grusas capers, the largest, can be up to ½ inch (12.7 mm) around. The term *caper berries* refers to the fully formed fruits, which are considered less desirable commercially. However, for home use, they are perfectly delicious.

To harvest, pick flower buds at the desired size or wait for the berries to plump. Rinse thoroughly, and layer fresh buds or berries in a jar with salt to preserve. Or place the buds or berries in a jar and cover with a 50/50 mix of 5 percent vinegar (e.g., apple cider or distilled vinegar) and water. Salt to taste. Pickle for 2 weeks before eating. Keep picked capers in the fridge or can in a water bath like vinegar pickles.

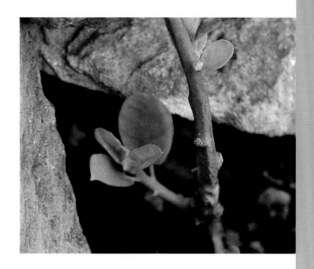

SPICE PROFILE
- **Names:** Caper, Caper Berry Bush
- **Latin:** *Capparis spinosa*
- **Native to:** Mediterranean (likely)
- **Edible parts:** Entire plant
- **Culinary uses:** Tangy flowers and berries are prepared as a condiment used in tapenades, sauces, soups, and with fish; leaves and roots are eaten and used in medicine

GROWING CONDITIONS
- Compact spreading or trailing habit; 2–3 feet (61–91 cm) tall and 3–6 feet (91–183 cm) wide
- Mature plant tolerance 25–105°F (-4–41°C); ideal growing range 55–85°F (13–30°C)
- Full sun, low-fertility, well-draining soil; pH 6.0–7.0
- 24+ months to harvest, self-fertile, cross-pollination recommended

ABOVE: *Each spring, capers will grow new stems and branches from the primary stem and crown area. It starts out spindly then becomes lush and abundant as it matures. You won't need to prune this plant to promote bushiness.*

MEDICINAL TIP

Many parts of the caper bush have been used as herbal remedies, including the root, leaves, fruits, and buds. In traditional Chinese medicine, caper fruits have been highlighted for their use treating degenerative arthritis.[28] This use has been verified in modern research, proving a capacity for decreasing inflammation and reducing pain signaling.[29] Experiment with this plant by using the leaves, buds, and berries in teas, tinctures (extraction by alcohol), or by eating fresh.

BAY LAUREL— A NOBLE SPICE

Is bay laurel a herb or a spice? Generally, herbs are the leafy parts of plants while spices are everything else. However, there is a school of spice thought that considers all semi-evergreen and evergreen plants to be spices.

These plants have more durable aromatic oils that enable longer term storage than soft-leaved herbs. That makes them more spicelike. Personally, I've included it because this book simply would not seem complete without it. It pairs well with nearly every other spice, especially for any meat or slow-cooking recipes.

Also, I love bay's associations with intellectual accomplishment. For example, baccalaureate— a word we use to denote completion of rigorous study—literally means "laurel berries." The titles "poet laureate" and "Nobel laureate" also pay homage to this tasty evergreen.

For those of you not content to rest on your laurels, and use bought bay, grow your own at home. Not only will it make your spice collection complete, but it can serve as a lovely reminder to keep learning about gardening and other noble pursuits.

Bay Laurel Care

Laurel is quite easy to grow if you give it lots of warmth and full sun. Frankly, other than adding compost annually, a monthly dousing with compost tea, and watering only when the top 2 inches (5 cm) of the soil dry out, this plant grows itself.

Since it has a shallow root system, wide rather than deep pots work best. Also, terracotta pots are great choice to improve drainage and prevent fungal pathogens for this drought-resistant plant.

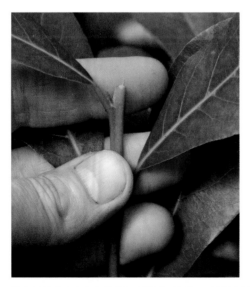 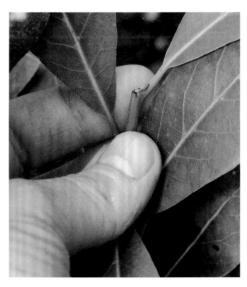

Make pruning cuts just above the secondary nodes near the leaf to promote upward growth (photo at left). If you cut into the secondary node, no branching will occur (photo at right). If you accidentally cut into the wrong place, just make fresh between the next set of leaves down.

Bay laurel can be trained as a tree or as a bush. To make it treelike, avoid trimming the growing tips until the plant has reached your desired height for it. Periodically remove unwanted stems and branches sprouting from the main trunk. Once the preferred height has been achieved, snip off the leaf tops to encourage more side-leafing and bushiness. To grow this plant as a bush, keep it compact by trimming the growing tips while the plant is young.

Harvesting

With bay, your prunings are your harvest. You can also collect individual leaves as needed. Dry leaves by laying them on a flat surface in a part of your kitchen where they'll remain dry. Or hang them by the stems. Once they're dry, seal them in a glass jar for several weeks to strengthen the aroma before using.

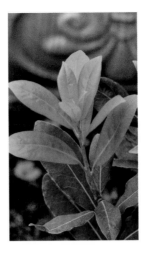 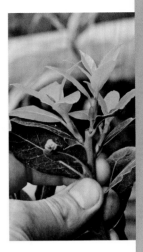

SPICE PROFILE
- **Names:** Sweet Bay, Bay laurel, Bay, Laurel
- **Latin:** *Laurus nobilis*
- **Native to:** Mediterranean and Asia Minor
- **Edible parts:** Oils in leaves
- **Culinary uses:** Savory leaf flavor enhances other herbs, spices, vegetables, and meats

GROWING CONDITIONS
- Plants grow 20–50 feet (6.1–15.2 m) in the ground, 6–10 feet (1.8–3 m) in containers
- Mature plant tolerance 27–80°F (-3–27°C); ideal temperature range 40–90°F (4–32°C)
- Full sun; fertile, well-draining soil; pH 6.0–7.0
- 18+ months to harvest; pollination not required for spice

MEDICINAL TIP

The magical leaf of the bay laurel plant has many medicinal applications, from increased digestion to antioxidant properties. It also has a history of ritualistic use in ceremonies of yore. This is likely due to its mild narcotic effects, as excessive leaf consumption can lead to an altered state of reality. The essential oils in this plant may expedite wound healing and reduce the risk of infection.[30] Make a strong tea and soak wounds in this solution to harness its beneficial actions.

ABOVE: *Notice the light-colored, newly formed leaves (photo at left). That new leaf segment is full of growth hormones. Prune the top section just above the first set of new leaves nearest to the old grow to cause branching (photo at right). This process is called "pinching" when applied to herbs.*

LAVENDER—
GROW FIELDS OF IT AT HOME

Lavender is often considered an herb. However, since you use the unopened flower buds, like capers, it can also be considered a spice. Also, like capers, some lavender loves growing under the Tuscan sun. Fields of it can be found in flowering in summer in those harsh, dusty Mediterranean soils.

Thankfully, you don't need to live in Tuscany, or even Provence, to create flowing fields of lavender at home. You just need to meet a few basic conditions and use cuttings to create a never-ending supply of lavender plants.

Lavender is one of the easiest spices to grow if you know four things.

1. Good drainage (rocks), some organic matter (compost), and low soil fertility (no fertilizer) are ideal for lavender production.

2. Prune the growing tips early and again after flowering to encourage branching and prevent plants from becoming woody.

3. Replace plants every 5 years.

4. Choose the right variety for your needs.

Points 1–3 are simple. Point number 4 is where most people go wrong. Many popular lavender landscape plants can only be grown as annuals in certain climates. Even if it says "perennial" on the plant tag, it may not be perennial in your climate. Choose varieties that are suited to your area's climate, humidity, and precipitation rates.

Also, select varieties based on their intended use. Some cultivars are best for perfume, others for culinary use, drying, or beauty products. There are over 450 known varieties of lavender. Take time to research and select the perfect plants for your needs and conditions.

Lavender is also the perfect plant to use to learn how to propagate cuttings. Cut a 3-inch (7.6 cm) leaf-covered stem segment from a live plant. Remove the bottom 1 inch of leaves. Place the cuttings in a shallow pot in moist potting soil. Keep in the sun, and water daily until roots form (4 weeks to 3 months).

When the roots form, pot up the cuttings. Begin pinching the growing tips every few weeks to promote branching. Plant outside in good weather or transplant to a larger pot.

With other plants, cutting propagation can be trickier. You may need to harvest from hard, semi-hard, or soft plant stems at different times of year. A rooting hormone might be required to expedite root formation. Moisture-loving plants also require high humidity to root from cuttings so covering with plastic may help.

Don't let those special conditions intimidate you. You're just taking few extra steps to create ideal microclimates for root development. That's no different than the skills used to grow exotic spices at home.

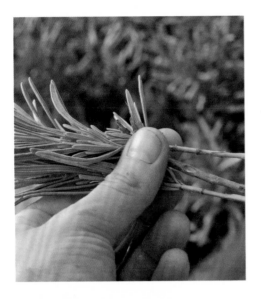

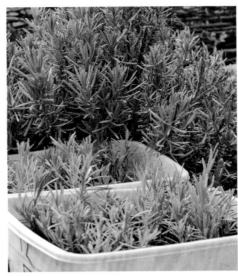

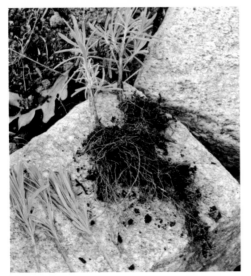

Don't worry if you rip the bark or cambium when removing leaves. That just makes the plants root faster. Also, you only need 2 inches (5 cm) of soil and about 1 inch (2.5 cm) of space per cutting. I use dollar store dishpans that have drilled drainage holes to make 20 cuttings at a time.

Herbes de Provence

Use the dried buds to make herbes de Provence. There's no set recipe, so feel free to experiment. Here's one of my favorites using dried herbs and spices that can be easily grown at home.

- 4 tablespoons (9.6 g) thyme
- 2 tablespoons (6 g) each of oregano, savory, rosemary
- 1 tablespoon (4.8 g) each of French tarragon, purple basil, and lavender buds
- Optional: ½ teaspoon (7.5 ml) ground fennel seeds

 MEDICINAL TIP

The anxiolytic, stress-reducing effects of lavender are undeniable. The next time you are feeling overwhelmed, and lavender is in bloom, spend a few minutes inhaling the aroma of your plants and evaluate how you feel afterward.

JUNIPER BERRY— THE HOMEGROWN CONE

I have a confession: I don't grow juniper at home anymore. I grow apples and juniper is a host for cedar apple rust. The disease is not lethal to either plant, but it's an additional stressor for apples, which already face fungal pathogens and climate volatility. Additionally, male junipers (required for pollination) produce so much pollen that you can see it in the air. That poses a problem for some allergy sufferers (such as me).

Despite those drawbacks, junipers are lovely, easy-to-grow landscape plants. They come in a variety of shapes and sizes from trees to prostrate shrubs.

Wild juniper is widely distributed across the Northern hemisphere. Unfortunately, wild juniper is also declining around the U.K. where most of the foraged juniper berries used to make gin grow. Low reproduction rates and fungal disease are the likely culprits for this decline. So if you love your London Dry, or botanical gins for that matter, planting juniper might be considered your civic duty.

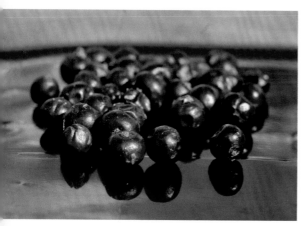

Dried juniper berries are often described as black or brown. Really, though, they look more like dark-colored rubies. This deep, dark, jewel-tone coloring is what to look for when drying juniper at home.

JUNIPER CARE
You can grow juniper in containers with sandy potting mixes. However, these plants will live longer (30-plus years) and have fewer problems if planted in low-fertility soils with excellent drainage. Rocky or sandy soil or fill dirt is best.

Loosen the soil in a planting area 3–4 times wider than the root mass. Incorporate compost to improve drainage and add nutrients. Water regularly until the plant begins actively growing. Then only water during extended droughts.

FINDING SPICE JUNIPERS
The big challenge with growing juniper is finding plants. You can start junipers from seed, but they might produce plants that are very different from their parent plants. Seedlings are also prone to death by unidentified causes. Start with 1-gallon plants or larger to save years of nursing seedlings to transplant size.

Most decorative landscape junipers are not cultivars of *Juniperus communis* used as a spice. Luckily, you can also use berries from cultivars of *Juniperus californica*, *Juniperus drupacea*, *Juniperus deppeana*, *Juniperus occidentalis*, and *Juniperus phoenicea* as spice. **Caution:** Other juniper varieties may be poisonous, and all juniper are poisonous in large quantities.

If the plant description mentions berries or cones, it's female. Males can be hard to find. Luckily, you may already have a male pollinizer nearby. Check online pollen trackers or ask your forestry office about juniper pollen prevalence to determine if you really need your own male pollinizer.

HARVESTING

Though they look like blueberries. juniper berries are small cones, botanically similar to pinecones. The cones form mostly in late spring. They develop fruit over a 6- to 18-month period, depending on variety.

Fruits are ready to harvest by picking when they develop that plump, dusky, blueberry appearance. Dry them on a flat surface until firm, but not fully desiccated. They turn purplish to blackish when they're dry.

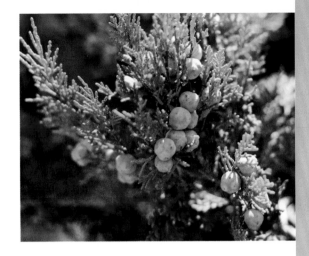

CULINARY TIP

Use juniper berries to make your own cordials by soaking a tablespoon or two in a bottle of brandy or vodka for a few weeks to extract the flavor. Add honey and rosemary to make it sweeter and more botanical tasting. Sieve and serve in a brandy snifter.

MEDICINAL TIP

Juniper has strong antimicrobial actions and can be burned like a sage bundle (berries and leaves alike) to volatilize its pathogen-busting components. Renowned for its use in urinary tract infections as an antiseptic due to its strong volatile oil content and ability to increase diuresis, juniper has been shown to decrease bacterial adhesion and reduce biofilm formation.[31] Caution is advised as too much juniper can be irritating to a body's tissues.

SPICE PROFILE

- **Name:** Common Juniper
- **Latin:** *Juniperus communis*
- **Native to:** Asia, Europe, and the United States
- **Edible parts:** Mature female cones
- **Culinary uses:** Astringent, piney, sweet flavor used for seasoning meat, fermented foods, pickles, and to make gin and juniper brandy

GROWING CONDITIONS

- Temperate climate, mature plant tolerance -40–85°F (4–29°C)
- Cold winters and comfortable summer climates are ideal
- Full sun to light shade, semi-dry to moist soil; pH 4.0–8.0
- 5+ years to harvest; male pollinizer required

ABOVE: *Junipers are an attractive evergreen plant that produces an edible and distinctly flavored berry-like cone.*

SUMAC—
LITTLE RED RHIZOME MAKER

Sumacs, *Rhus coriaria*, are stunning, compact, leguminous trees that grow well in poor-quality or rocky soils. The fruits, called *drupes*, have soft outer skins, fleshy interiors, and central seeds. Though smaller in size, the fruit structure is just like a peach. The pericarps, or the fleshy part and skin outside the seeds, are used as spice.

Ground sumac pericarps provide the dominant taste profile in Mediterranean za'atar and Egyptian dukkah spice mixes. Its lemony, tangy, and slightly starchy flavor also works well in meat rubs.

Rhus coriaria is commonly used for commercial spice production. It requires Mediterranean climate conditions to survive. However, temperate varieties such as smooth sumac (*Rhus glabra*) and staghorn sumac (*Rhus typhina*) have edible fruits that can be used as a substitute.

These plants spread by rhizomes underground and over long distances in loose, shallow soil. They are often considered invasive due to their fast-growing, easy-spreading habits. Keep sumac in check by creating underground, non-permeable permanent root perimeters as you would for bamboo.

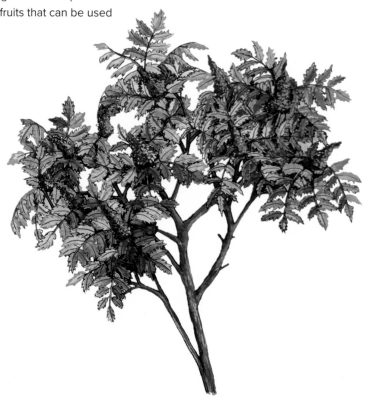

If sumac does escape your barrier, don't mow it down. Instead, peel the bark around the tree, as if you were air layering, but don't wrap it. This prevents the adult plant from storing nutrients in its rhizomes and spreading. (It also ultimately kills a tree, so use this only on unwanted plants.)

The Latin word *rhus* means "red." All edible sumacs have red drupes when fully ripe (though not all red sumacs are tasty). Former members of the *Rhus* species, that have now been reclassified include poison ivy (*Toxicodendron radicans*), poison oak (*Toxicodendron diversilobum*), and poison sumac (*Toxicodendron vernix*). These allergy-causing plants have whitish drupes and can be easily distinguished from edible sumacs by their fruit color.

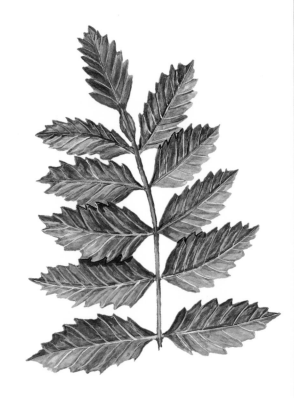

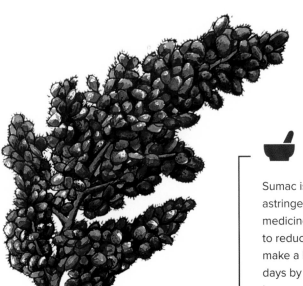

MEDICINAL TIP

Sumac is one of herbalism's great astringents. It's traditionally used in folk medicine of the Southern United States to reduce excessive sweating. You can make a lovely lemonade for hot summer days by sun-infusing sumac berries and lemons, and then adding honey to taste.

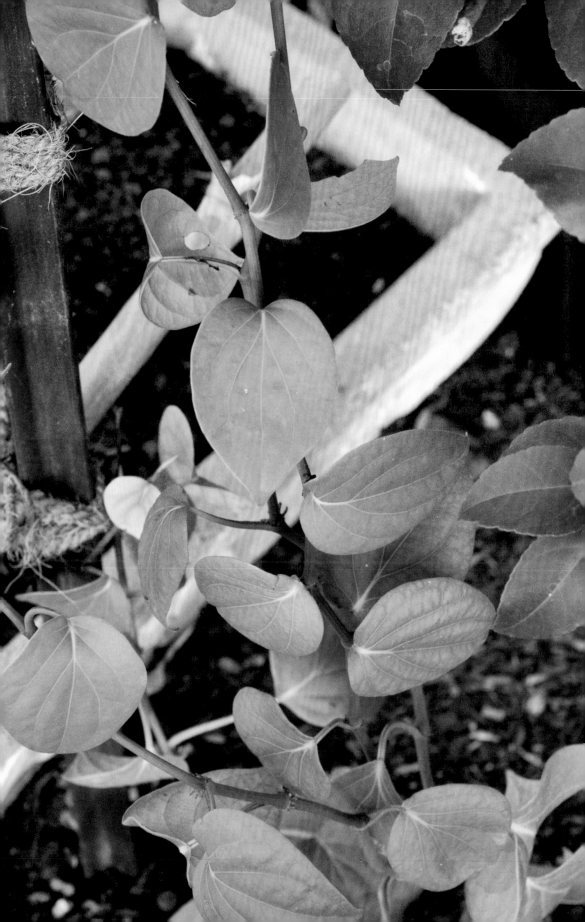

TROPICAL AND SUBTROPICAL CLIMATE PERENNIAL SPICES

The spices in this section cannot tolerate cold temperatures. You will need to provide consistently warm temperatures year-round. They also require higher levels of humidity than temperate or Mediterranean plants.

ANNATTO OR ACHIOTE	**98**
ALLSPICE	**100**
CINNAMON	**102**
VANILLA	**106**
TAMARIND	**109**
PEPPERCORN	**110**
CLOVE, NUTMEG, STAR ANISE	**112**

< Given that black pepper was once valued more highly than gold, you'd expect this plant to be hard to grow at home. Actually, though, it's quite easy, even in small pots. You just need a bit of patience and a mostly sunny to partly shady spot and room for the vine trellis to stand up.

ANNATTO OR ACHIOTE— A CELEBRATION OF COLOR

In the U.S., many of us grew up on "white bread culture." This means we eat a lot of bland, highly processed foods. Our main spices consist of salt and black pepper. In this context, achiote seems like an exotic spice. Yet it's found on many sandwiches made with white bread. That's because, under the name *annatto*, it gives American and cheddar cheeses their signature orange color.

In cheese, this pasty, slightly sweet and piquant substance saturates with color. It also binds milk fats in a tighter "knit," making the resulting cheese stick to your teeth and taste buds. This is achiote's true power. It thickens to enhance mouthfeel and gives other flavors more staying power.

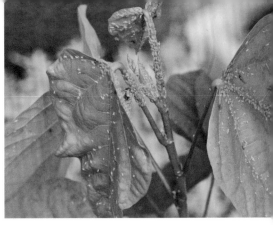

Indoor and greenhouse-raised annatto seems to be a favorite of aphids. Use soapy water to wipe them away or remove infested leaves.

I imagine that's why it's a key ingredient in the famous graveside gourmet delicacy called Mucbipollo (buried chicken). This traditional Mexican dish is served as an offering to the deceased and the living on Día de los Muertos (Day of the Dead). Undoubtedly, during the lengthy and ritualistic preparation of this celebratory dish, the rich red color of achiote serves as vivid visual indicator of the blood that binds us to our ancestors and descendants.

For me, achiote reminds me of my childhood in Southern California when I ate American cheese sandwiches and achiote-colored Mexican rice. I also colored on the sidewalk with achiote seeds scavenged from a neighbor's yard.

As a garden meditation, this spice's importance on Day of the Dead and the delicate heartlike leaves remind me that love is something we can all freely give that transcends even the grave.

ANNATTO CARE

Annatto requires warm temperatures and full sun for heavy fruit production. When those conditions are met, it's easy to grow. This showy spice plant is beautiful for use on a summer patio or in your greenhouse. In warm climates it can also be planted as an interesting evergreen hedge.

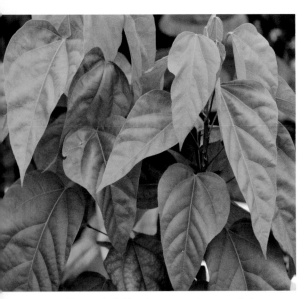

The slight fold in the center gives annatto's tear-shaped leaves the impression of being heart-shaped. Understory leaves may get shaded out by bushy top growth. You can remove any discolored leaves as needed to maintain the decorative beauty of your annatto.

Soil depth, rather than width, is key for this taprooted plant. It works well in modern-style tall and narrow planters. Although it can become a large tree, it's typically top-pruned to control its size or coppiced to make it a shrub. (See page 105 for directions on how to coppice to create multiple trunks.)

Annatto is most prolific in organic matter rich soil. Water deeply only when the top couple inches of soil are dry to encourage deep rooting.

This plant is partially self-fertile. For best yields, though, you'll need cross-pollination and a thriving bee population.

Fertility needs are minimal. Add compost annually. Water potted plants with compost tea monthly while plants are actively growing.

HARVESTING

Annatto's summer flowers give way to spiky burrs. These turn bright red and then fade to brown as they dry over a 3- to 4-month period into fall. When the burrs crack at their tips, harvest the entire fruit. Pry open the pod to remove the seeds.

Dried seeds can be ground and powdered using a high-quality seed grinder. Or they can be used to infuse oil or water. To infuse, warm 1 cup (235 ml) of liquid for every ¼ cup (60 ml) of seeds. Heat slowly over a low flame. Avoid boiling to prevent bitterness.

For use in home cheesemaking, add seeds when pasteurizing your milk. When the desired color is reached, strain the liquid through a sieve. Or add annatto-infused water with your rennet.

Some herbal medicine recipes and industrial applications call for alcohol, glycerite, or vinegar extractions. In those cases, heating is not necessary and the liquid to seed ratio varies by application.

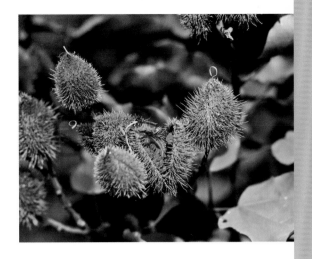

SPICE PROFILE
- **Names:** Annatto, Achiote, Lipstick Tree
- **Latin:** *Bixa orellana*
- **Native to:** Tropical parts of Mexico, and Central and South America
- **Edible parts:** Seeds
- **Culinary use:** Mild pasty flavor used as a natural food color, and spice mix thickener

GROWING CONDITIONS
- Tropical and subtropical; grows to 10–30 feet (3–9.1 m) in ground, 5–8 feet (1.5–2.4 m) in containers
- Mature plant tolerance 35–100°F (2–38°C); ideal temperature range 60–85°F (16–29°C)
- Full sun; organic matter, rich, well-draining soil; pH 6.0–7.5
- 2+ years to harvest, cross-pollination recommended

ABOVE: *Annatto produces spiky burrs that crack open when the seeds inside are ready to harvest.*

ALLSPICE— AN UNEXPECTED HARVEST

Warning! Many attempts to raise these trees outside their native regions have resulted in lush, lovely plants that produce nearly no fruit. However, let me explain why you might still want to take a risk on allspice.

The fruiting habits of allspice is one of nature's many mysteries. Some of the literature suggests that there are distinctly male and female plants. But based on the accounts I've read, the term nonbinary better captures the full reproductive diversity found in allspice populations.

There are allspice plants with female flowers that do not produce fruit even when they're pollinated by a male pollinizer. There are plants that appear to have primarily female flowers that produce abundant fruit even without a male pollinizer. There are plants with predominantly male flowers that sometimes spontaneously produce fruit. In other words, allspice can't be uniformly categorized into easy-to-check boxes.

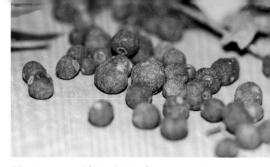

Allspice—named for its hints of cinnamon, clove, nutmeg, black pepper, and vanilla—has fragrant, edible leaves and (sometimes) berries that can be used fresh or dried in cooking, tea making, and in potpourri.

It all comes down to a kind of genetic lottery. Allspice don't fruit until they are about 7 years old. So the general practice in Jamaica (where 90 percent of the world's allspice is grown) has been to plant three plants from seed together in a patch. After 7 years, those that produce allspice fruits are kept. Some non-producing plants with mostly male flowers are also kept for cross-pollination. The remaining non-producers are culled to give the keepers space to grow 30 feet (9.1 m) tall.

Vegetative reproduction of the fruit-bearing trees has also been in practice since 1960s. Air layering and grafting (growing a cutting of a productive plant on another plant's roots) have produced good results. However, nursery production has been erratic and grafted or cloned plants are hard to come by. As such, most planters still rely on the "plant three, wait and see" approach to growing allspice.

There are also benefits to favoring this kind of genetic gambling. The plants kept for spice tend to be healthy, hardy, and easy to care for. Continuously cloning the same few plants mean all of those clones could be at risk for mass die offs from a single disease or pathogen. The global banana supply, for example, is currently facing this problem. Genetic diversity, by contrast, ensures production security.

So although allspice berries aren't guaranteed, if you start plants from seed, you might just win the genetic lottery. You can improve

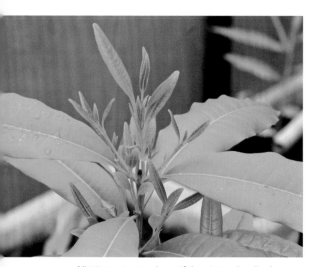

Allspice puts on a beautiful spring color display as its tiny leaves open with dark bronze hues and grow rapidly to large-sized lobes.

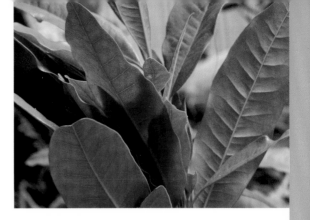

MEDICINAL TIP

Dried allspice berries provide a sweet and spicy taste to herbal formulas and can be used as a corrigent, a flavoring agent to make medicines taste more palatable. Medicinally, allspice is employed as an anti-infective remedy to reduce respiratory infections, and the congestion associated with them.[32] Make a cup of hot tea with the ground berries to use this medicine.

SPICE PROFILE
- **Names:** Allspice, Jamaica Pepper, Myrtle Pepper, Pimento
- **Latin:** *Pimenta dioica*
- **Native to:** West Indies and Central America
- **Edible parts:** Unripe fruits and leaves
- **Culinary uses:** All-in-one spice flavor used in jerk seasoning, soup, sauces, pickling, fermented meats, desserts, and liqueurs

your chances by planting three seed-started trees. Or you can talk someone with a fruit-bearing allspice into making you a clone and a male pollinizer for best results.

Even if you never get berries, allspice leaves are deliciously aromatic and can be used like bay leaves in cooking and teas. Plus, these plants are lovely, fragrant, and easy to grow in containers.

GROWING CONDITIONS
- Mature plant tolerance 35–80°F (2–27°C); ideal temperature range 55–85°F (13–29°C)
- Full sun or light shade; fertile, moist soil; pH 6.0–7.0
- 7+ years to harvest; male pollinizer recommended

ALLSPICE CARE

Allspice plants are quite undemanding. Keeping them in temperatures above freezing is a must. Grow them in a large tree pot with a good potting soil mix. Water when the soil feels dry in the top 2 inches (5 cm). Apply compost tea weekly during the growing season and, monthly when leaf production slows. Top off compost annually. Then wait for 7+ years to see if you've got a winning plant.

ABOVE: *Allspice is enigmatic plant with difficult-to-categorize flowering habits. Producing fruit is not a straightforward prospect. Thankfully, its abundant leaves are an aromatic, edible alternative.*

HARVESTING ALLSPICE

Use your pruned leaves as your harvest or remove individual leaves as you need them. If your plant produces berries, harvest when they're fully formed and barely beginning to flush with a hint of nongreen color. Air dry, and then use whole or powdered. Ripe, fresh fruits can also be used.

Bonus! If you can grow allspice, you can also grow bay rum (*Pimenta racemosa*) as another lovely plant for your spice and fragrance garden.

CINNAMON—
A TRULY
WONDERFUL WEED

Cinnamon is an invasive weed. Its seeds self-sow. Young plants grow quickly in low-fertility soil and in the shade of other plants. In the Seychelle Islands, for example, the indigenous fruit pigeon and the Indian mynah birds eat the seeds and disperse them among other vegetation. Rain beats the seeds into the ground and warm conditions expedite germination. Then cinnamon's natural ability to thrive in low-fertility soil and shade give it a competitive edge over other plants.

Unfortunately for spice lovers, cinnamon only grows like a weed in regions with consistently warm temperatures of around 80°. Most of us have to do a little work to stimulate the perfect microclimate and growing conditions for cinnamon to thrive.

Brown leaf tips typically indicate insufficient water and they can also be a sign of boggy soil. Check soil drainage and water consistently. With good care, most plants can recover. Sometimes, especially in young plants, this can indicate severe heat stress that has led to systemic failure of the plant's ability to uptake water and nutrients.

Also, for a continuous harvest, you'll need to grow your own cinnamon more like it is grown in its native lands of Sri Lanka. There it's coppiced and cared for much like a vineyard or orchard. Precise cultivation and a bit of constructive stress have made Sri Lankan-grown cinnamon the most prized in the world.

CINNAMON CARE

I read that cinnamon was easy to grow as a potted plant. Ironically, it's the only spice I've had challenges growing. I started with a 2-inch (5 cm) potted tissue clone sent by mail during a heat wave. The plant arrived, inside a box, inside a plastic bag full of water droplets. I knew before I opened the bag that the poor plant's chances of survival were miniscule.

Technically, plants don't sweat, they *transpire*. Yet the process is similar to how we cool ourselves by sweating. Plants drink water through their roots. The water flows through the xylem in the stem, up to the leaves, where it escapes through small pores called *stomas*. Then the water vapor on the leaf surfaces evaporates, thereby cooling the plant.

All those droplets in the bag meant my plant had been transpiring like crazy. But since all that heat and moisture were trapped in plastic, there was no way my juvenile cinnamon had been able to stay cool. Like humans in excessive humidity, plants are at greater risk for heat stroke. Also like us, when this happens, critical life support systems fail quickly. Roots and leaves die, photosynthesis stops, water and nutrient uptake shuts down, and the plant becomes sickly or dies.

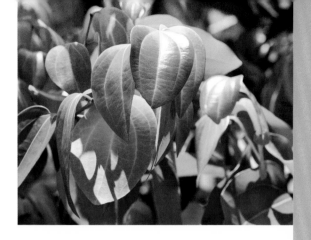

Mature cinnamon is adapted to grow extremely well at temperatures just above 80°F (27°C) even with relative humidity levels of around 80 percent. However, since young cinnamon is adapted to grow in the shade of other plants, they have much lower heat and humidity thresholds than older plants. The soil they thrive in is cooled and kept moist by adjacent plants. They also receive the cooling benefits of those older, more established plants that are transpiring. Growing in the shadow of a bigger tree is like standing next to an air conditioner vent for cinnamon.

As I expected, my poor little overly packaged plant never thrived as it should have. I tell you this tale not as discouragement, but as a lesson as to why it's important to nurse young plants carefully. Also, it's a good reminder that even plants adapted to hot conditions must be able to transpire so they don't expire.

Thankfully, most cinnamon plants will grow with no problems if you follow these simple steps.

1. Order your plants for delivery during ideal weather. To the best of your ability, check the weather forecast all along the most likely path for delivery to ensure plants won't get too hot or too cold in transit.

2. Plant it in a potting mix that includes sand, aged compost, and leaf mold or peat moss to promote drainage. If you can get the pH to be around 5.5, that's even better.

3. Add compost annually to simulate the natural addition of decomposed matter that occurs naturally in a forest ecosystem.

4. Give it consistent warmth between 65–80°F (18–29°C) with a fair amount of humidity.

5. Water regularly, but don't allow the soil to become waterlogged.

SPICE PROFILE
- **Names:** Cinnamon, True cinnamon, Ceylon Cinnamon
- **Latin:** *Cinnamomum verum* (syn. *innamomum zeylanicum*)
- **Native to:** Sri Lanka
- **Edible parts:** Bark, leaves, fruits
- **Culinary uses:** Spicy, sweet, musky flavor used for desserts, curries, soups, rubs, marinades, mole sauce

GROWING CONDITIONS
- Tropical and subtropical; can be a tree or coppiced shrub; 5–8 feet (1.5–2.4 m) tall in containers
- Mature plant tolerance 40–95°F (4–35°C);
  ideal temperature range 65–85°F (18–29°C)
- Full sun to part shade
- Low fertility; organic matter; rich, moist soil; pH 4.5–6.5
- Typically started from seed, cuttings, or tissue clones
- 24+ months to harvest
- Cross-pollination unnecessary for bark production

ABOVE: *The foliage of cinnamon plants is glossy green, with new growth often tinged with red.*

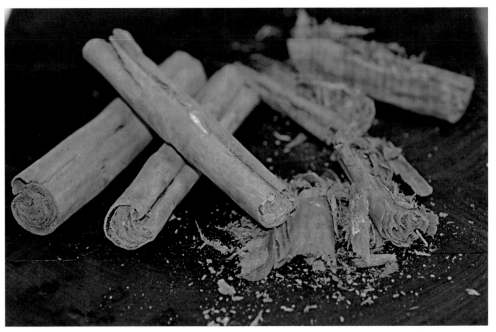

Commercially grown cinnamon is harvested in long strips, rolled in bunches, and then cut to size. At home, you don't have to be as tidy with your strips or drying techniques as those extremely skilled professionals.

6. Keep young plants in part shade with moist roots (in the company of other plants if possible) until they have enough top growth to shade their own roots.

7. Gradually move cinnamon plants toward full sun conditions as they mature.

8. Pot up to larger pots as needed, especially if you coppice your tree for a larger harvest.

Learning about cinnamon reminded of an important gardening lesson: Weeds are just plants grown in the wrong place. The next time you come across a weed you don't know, think of cinnamon. Then do a little research to identify that plant out of place. You might discover something useful growing like a "weed" in your own backyard.

HARVESTING

The entire cinnamon plant is edible. However, the inner bark is prized as spice. When your tree is about 3 years old and in good health, coppice the tree. To coppice, cut the trunk down to a few inches from the ground. Make the cut on an angle so water runs off. Soon after cutting, multiple trunks will grow from the root clump.

The harvested trunk is your first cinnamon bark harvest. In future years, harvest a few of the coppiced trunks at a time, always leaving some behind to continue growing.

To peel the bark, use a knife to scrape the exterior bark layer off the trunk. Then use a knife to cut out a section of the inner bark so you can begin to score and peel the inner

CINNAMON VS. CASSIA

*C*innamomum cassia, referred to just as "cinnamon" in the U.S. and as "cassia" in other countries, is a close cousin to *Cinnamomum verum*. The two plants grow in similar conditions. Yet cassia's bark is much harder to remove and can't be ground using inexpensive spice grinders.

Cinnamomum burmanni and *Cinnamomum loureiroi* are close relatives with similar growth habits but different taste profiles.

bark from the trunk. You can stack layers of inner bark on to each other and allow them to curl and dry together. Then cut them to a manageable length to give them the appearance of the cinnamon quills sold at stores.

If you prefer not to coppice your tree into a bush, you can also just harvest the whips. Whips are the young stems and branches under 2 years of age that can be similarly peeled or used whole. Your yields will be reduced, but your tree can be kept more compact.

The leaves and fruits can also be used for oil distillations or as aromatic agents in things such as potpourri.

MEDICINAL TIP

Upon consumption, cinnamon imparts both mucilaginous and astringent medicinal properties. The demulcent activity of cinnamon reigns supreme in diabetic conditions. Taken in larger doses, cinnamon is shown to significantly reduce glucose and triglyceride levels, making it an effective medicinal ally for diabetes.[33] For sore throats the demulcent, astringent, and antimicrobial actions of cinnamon can be put to use by mixing it with honey to reduce irritation.

VANILLA—
THE INIMITABLE

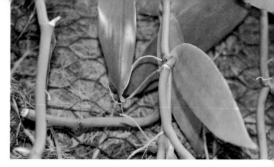

In the aviary at the North Carolina Zoo, a very long vanilla plant grows in an up-and-down zig-zag pattern along a wall lined with coconut coir and chicken wire. Some of the aerial roots attach to the coconut fiber and grow, while others that don't find traction wither.

Despite its enduring, exotic mystique, vanilla is well-suited to being kept as a house orchid or conservatory plant. It only requires these six things to grow well:

1. forest litter
2. appropriate trellising
3. indirect sunlight
4. consistent moisture
5. constant warmth
6. hand-pollination

Hand-pollination is the most challenging of these criteria to meet. Though the process is simple, it must be performed daily for about two months starting in early spring. Flowers form in clusters along the length of the vine, with only one or two flowers per cluster opening each day at sunrise.

To hand-pollinate, carefully remove the flower petals, leaving the reproductive column intact. Find the rostellum, which is a hooked flap that protects the pollinia, or clusters of pollen, that sit loosely atop the anther lobes.

Now, here's where nature gets tricky. Just below that flap is less obvious flap called a *labellum*. The labellum hides the stigma, effectively making it impossible for vanilla to self-pollinate.

Using a toothpick, gently raise the labellum flap while gently pressing the pollinia-covered anthers into the stigma using the rostellum flap. It sounds complicated, but it's a bit like pushing the opening flap of an envelope inside the letter pocket. (See illustration on page 108.)

When grown in its native habitat, Melipona bees, and occasionally other orchid bees, hummingbirds, and even crickets, can pollinate vanilla. Everywhere else on earth, humans handle the pollination. It's important to note that the self-fertile flowers will produce vanilla pods. But only cross-pollinated flowers will produce viable seeds. Unless you intentionally cross-pollinate multiple vanilla plants, propagate new plants using 8- to 12-inch (20–30 cm) cuttings from a mature vine.

As for those other five requirements, plant your vanilla in orchid soil mix. Or go into the woods and gather up bark, leaves, and some forest soil as your potting medium. Moss can also be used to help retain moisture. (Of course, harvest sustainably and only with permission.)

Put your planting medium in a 3- to 5-gallon (11.4–19 L) pot. Or create your own bark-lined container using chicken wire, twine, and a little creativity.

In order to trellis vanilla, it must grow at least 3–5 feet (91–152 cm) tall and then grow downward to flower. After this, it can grow in a zig zag pattern, up and down, for lengths of 30 feet (9.1 m) or more. You can trim it to keep it closer to 15 feet (4.6 m). Fruiting will occur mostly on the downward-growing vines.

Technically, any trellising that allows enough vertical height and width and will support the weight of the plant will do. For metal, plastic, wood, or bamboo trellising, you'll need to tie the vanilla vine to the trellis. Alternatively, you can grow the vine up other trees or on trellises covered with bark to offer the aerial roots organic matter they can attach themselves to.

In nature, vanilla is an understory plant. This vining orchid grows up the trunks of sturdy trees, receiving the filtered sunlight that splays through the leaves. It's an epiphytic plant, not a parasitic plant, so it uses its host as a trellis without doing harm to the tree.

Aerial roots, located under each vanilla leaf, adhere to textured bark. Just like underground roots, aerial roots act like anchors to fix the vine in place. They also absorb moisture and nutrients from minuscule bits of decaying matter on bark surfaces. You can even grow vanilla on the trunk of your container-grown tropical or subtropical spice trees if you give them a head start to gain height before training the vanilla.

Those adventitious aerial roots also make starting new vanilla plants from cuttings extra easy. This is typically how they are propagated commercially. Sellers sometimes send unrooted vanilla cuttings for you to root at home. Cuttings that are 8 inches (20 cm) long take 3–4 years to reach flowering maturity. Longer cuttings may flower faster.

Due to its natural growth habit, vanilla makes a wonderful choice for an indoor vertical plant wall with other filtered light loving epiphytes such as ferns. You can also train vanilla over smooth surfaces such as metal or bamboo, but you'll need to use ties to hold the vines up.

Always protect vanilla vines from direct sunlight either by careful positioning or using shade cloth. Keep your vanilla plant above 60°F (16°C) in winter. Aim for 75°F (24°C) or above from spring to fall. Keep the potting mix moist but never boggy. Mist leaves and aerial roots twice a day during dry periods. During flowering and fruiting, keep humidity above 50 percent. Use a humidifier or keep a pot of water near the base of the plant to maintain moisture in the air.

HARVESTING AND CURING PODS

Pods form a few weeks after pollination and will take 7–8 months to mature. Harvest

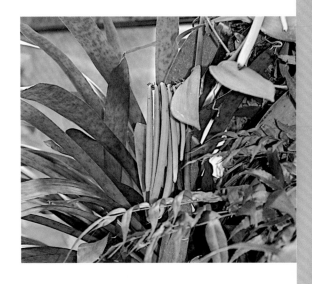

SPICE PROFILE
- **Names:** Vanilla, Bourbon/Madagascar Vanilla, Tahitian Vanilla
- **Latin:** *Vanilla planifolia*
- **Native to:** Mexico
- **Edible parts:** Fruit pods
- **Culinary uses:** Sweet, aromatic used in desserts, and baked goods

GROWING CONDITIONS
- Mature plant tolerance 50–90°F (10–32°C); ideal temperature range 70–85°F (21–29°C)
- Indirect, filtered light; organic matter; rich, moist soil; pH 6.0–7.0
- 3+ years to harvest; hand-pollination required

ABOVE: *At the North Carolina Zoo, ready-to-harvest vanilla pods hang like green beans from this tropical vining orchid. Like the nearby ferns, this spice is an epiphyte that naturally grows on other plants without causing parasitic harm.*

when the tips begin to yellow but before they split. Blanch the pods in boiling water for 1 minute to prevent further ripening.

Wrap the pods in a thick towel or felted wool fabric and store them in a very warm location to sweat them. Once a day, remove the pods from the towel and expose them to hot sun for a few hours to dry surface moisture and prevent mold. Then rewrap them and return them to their warm location. Repeat this process for 7 days. The goal is to create internal fermentation before intensive drying begins.

After the sweating, dry the pods in sun to part sun for 3 weeks or until about one-third of the original moisture level. In wet climates, you can do this in your turned-off oven with the light left on for heat. During drying the vanilla beans should develop their characteristic vanilla flavor. After drying, store those pods in a warm, dry location for another 6 months or more to allow the flavor to fully develop before using.

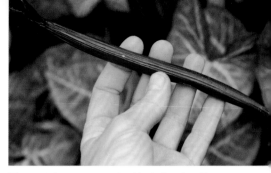

This pod, from a vine at the North Carolina Zoo, is past its peak for spice production. The tip is split and it's fully ripe. At home, harvest pods with just a hint of yellow at the top and before the pods split.

 MEDICINAL TIP

Vanilla's familiar taste and aroma can make your mouth water. As such, it can help increase appetites.[34] Topically, vanilla can be used as a soothing treatment for irritation of tissues and is a folk remedy for treating burns. To make a topical vanilla oil, place chopped vanilla bean pods in a carrier oil, such as almond or grapeseed, and let them macerate to extract the medicine.

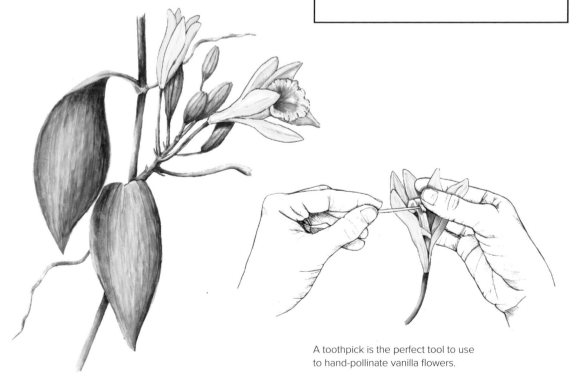

A toothpick is the perfect tool to use to hand-pollinate vanilla flowers.

TAMARIND AND THE ART OF BONSAI

Tamarind (*Tamarindus indica*) is basically a bean tree. It's a legume, like fenugreek, and fixes its own nitrogen in collaboration with rhizobia. In the ground it can grow slowly to 100 feet (30 m) tall with a trunk 25 feet (7.6 m) wide. However, tamarind also grows well as a bonsai. It can even produce a fair amount of spice at only a few feet tall.

To grow tamarind as a beloved bonsai, start a few seeds in full sun in a shallow pot or buy a young plant. When the tree is about 2 feet (61 cm) tall and growing well, use a fork to carefully scrape the soil from the roots. Trim any downward-growing anchor roots to be even with the lateral roots. Then replant your tamarind in a shallow bonsai pot, using bonsai soil mix (available online or at garden supply stores).

Trim the growing tips of your tree to keep it short and make it bushier. Leave all side branches until the plant recovers from the root trimming and repotting. Thereafter, trim as needed to control for size and shape. Grow tamarind trees in full sun or bright, indirect sunlight such as through a south-facing window.

Potted tamarind require regular watering. Monthly applications of liquid bonsai fertilizer during the growing season are encouraged. Repot in new bonsai soil mix, and a slightly larger pot, every few years.

Tamarinds are partially self-fertile but require insect pollination. Hand-pollination is also effective. Grow two bonsai tamarinds to cross-pollinate for better yields.

At about 6 years of age, healthy tamarinds (even tiny ones) can produce abundant fruits that are very much like large bean pods. You can eat these fresh like an apple, turn the pulp into a paste, or dry the pods and grind all but the skin into a powder. Immature fruits are sour, but more mature fruits are sweeter. Time your harvest according to your taste preference and cooking needs.

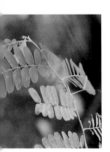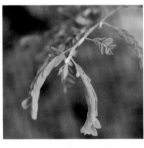

Tamarind leaves open during the day and close as dusk approaches. This lovely, restful habit makes it an interesting addition to an indoor container garden. You'll just need to keep this otherwise giant tree compact using bonsai techniques.

PEPPERCORNS— THE HELEN OF SPICE

Some call it the king of spice, but I think of it as the "Helen of Spice." After all, this potent pea-sized prize literally launched thousands of ships to sail from Europe through open waters to the Malabar coast of India and elsewhere. Battles have been fought and fortunes made and lost, over this one, beautifully enigmatic, irreplaceable spice.

Once upon a time, black pepper held more value than gold and was even a preferred currency in times of turbulence. Today it's considered ordinary and is as taken for granted as table salt. No longer locked in chests and valued like money, we even dispense it from disposable containers while eating in our cars.

More than any other spice, pepper makes it clear exactly how much our human priorities have changed. If I were to compare its

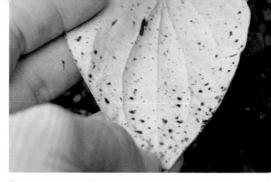

The undersides of black pepper leaves, especially if the plant is grown in more lighted conditions, form mineral deposits called *exudates*. They're completely normal and don't harm the plant.

historical value to something similar today, it would be similar to platinum, cobalt, or lithium, which are used in technologies deemed critical to our lives today.

BLACK PEPPER CARE

Though it's not an orchid, pepper grows much like vanilla. It has aerial roots that cling to live or decaying tree bark. These multistemmed vines can be trained on other trees or over other kinds of trellising. They can grow to 30 feet (9.1 m) tall but will fruit even if pruned to a few feet in length.

Pepper production starts when plants are about 3–5 years and reaches full production at around 7 years.

Plants grown in too little light have small dark leaves and low fruit production. However, that fruit may be more pungent and powerful. In full sun or indirect sun, the leaves are larger, lighter green on top and nearly yellow underneath. They can look almost unhealthy, with occasional black speckled nutrient deposits on the undersides. Yet these slightly stressed plants produce abundant berry clusters that start in summer and are ready to harvest in 6–8 months.

Piper nigrum is believed to be self-fertile though it will be more productive when wind or insect pollinated. At the North Carolina Zoo, even in a greenhouse, the pepper spikes were mostly pollinated without any special effort. But if you move your plant outdoors when the flower spikes appear, or

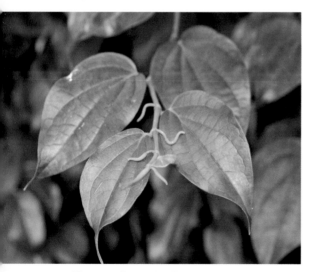

Those small, wormlike flower spikes are the start of pepper production. If the plant is mature, after pollination, the spikes will elongate and fatten into cylindrical pepper clusters. When a pepper plant is grown in shade, as it is in this photo taken at the North Carolina Zoo, the spikes often shrivel without producing fruit.

MEDICINAL TIP

Black pepper is not only one of the most sought-after spices, but it's a strong medicine as well. Researched for its antioxidant, analgesic, and neuroprotective effects, its medicinal potential is great.[35] However, it can also increase the bioavailability of medicinal phytochemicals by consuming it with other plants, such as turmeric.[36] Add extra black pepper to all your spice-rich foods and drinks to increase their medicinal activities.

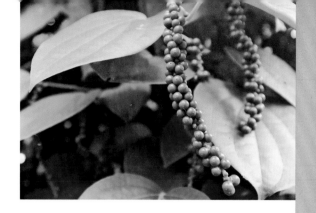

SPICE PROFILE
- **Names:** Black Pepper, Peppercorns
- **Latin:** *Piper nigram*
- **Native to:** Malabar, India
- **Edible parts:** Entire plant is edible
- **Culinary uses:** Spicy, burning, hot mustard taste used for sushi

GROWING CONDITIONS
- Subtropical, mature plant tolerance 45–95°F (7–35°C); ideal temperature range 65–85°F (18–29°C)
- Full sun to part shade; fertile, moist soil; pH 6.0–7.0
- 5+ years to harvest; aelf-fertile/ cross-pollination

ABOVE: *Black pepper grows on long vines and was once more valuable than gold.*

use a fan to simulate wind, pollination might be improved. The pollen and stigmas are believed to be viable for 3–4 days and possibly, up to 10 days.

Water regularly and mist vines during dry periods. Increase humidity when the flower spikes appear until fruit forms to improve productivity.

HARVESTING

Black, white, green, and red peppercorns (also called berries) come from the same plant. Harvest black peppercorns in clusters like grapes when they're plump and fully formed but still green. Gather them in a breathable bag, such as burlap, and allow them to warm up and ferment or sweat (like vanilla) for a day or two. Then remove the stems. Lay the berries on a dark tarp in direct sun or put them on a sheet pan in a 100–120° (38–93°C) oven. Turn them periodically until they dry to a dark brown or blackish. Green peppercorns are harvested at the same time as the black but are preserved in vinegar (like capers) to keep them tender.

White peppercorns are harvested slighter later than black ones. Traditionally, the berries are placed in running water for a week or

more to soften the pericarps, or outer skins, so they can be easily removed. At home, you can boil your berries for 15 minutes until the skins are pliant. Allow the skins to cool, then rub them off between your fingers. Dry the inner portions in direct sunlight to lighten the color and mellow the flavor.

Red peppercorns are ripened on the plant and then harvested and dried.

FOR REAL RISK TAKERS:
CLOVE, NUTMEG, STAR ANISE

When you're ready to add a few more spices to your repertoire, other classics such as clove, nutmeg, and star anise are worth considering. Plants and viable seeds can be hard to find. Also, these aren't as well-suited to container growing as the other tropical/subtropical spices in this section. Yet if you have a large greenhouse or conservatory, or live in the tropics, these might be worth a try. Here's some information to get you started in your research.

Cloves (*Syzygium aromaticum*) are the easiest of these three long-term-commitment spices. They can be started from freshly harvested seeds and cuttings. They can be kept in tree-sized pots using a potting mix with lots of organic matter.

Fruit production begins as early as 6 years after planting but takes 15 years or more to reach full production. Also, the plants often will not survive to full production in a

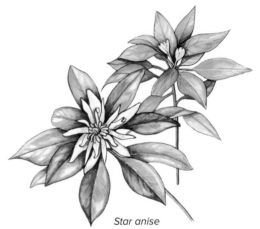

Star anise

container. You may be able get some fruit production before the plant requires more space than is reasonable to provide in a pot.

Cloves are self-fertile so you will only need one plant. For good production, insect cross-pollination is considered necessary. Take your plants outdoors during flowering. Hand-pollination is also possible, but it's not commonly used.

Nutmeg (*Myristica fragrans*) is a large tree that needs warm weather, preferably above 75°F (24°C). Female plants produce fruit and a male pollinizer is required for spice production. Plants started from seed tend to be about half male and half female. Unfortunately, plant sex can't be determined until flowering which begins at about 8 years

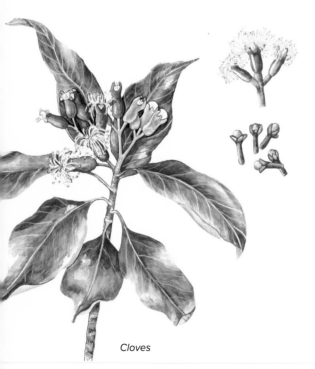

Cloves

of age. Starting with sexed plants propagated by cloning, layering, or cuttings is best to ensure pollination. Trees reach full production at about 25 years of age.

At food stores you'll normally only find nutmeg, which is the inner-seed portion of the fruit. Sometimes you can find dried ground mace, which comes from the red aril wrapped around the nutmeg seed. When you grow this at home, you can also use the outer pericarp fruit and skin to make fragrant candies and jams.

Star anise (*Illicium vernum*) is a lovely tree or shrub with fragrant flowers and star-shaped fruits. The fruits are harvested when they're fully plump but still green. They are dried whole. The glossy inner seeds have the most intense flavor, but the entire fruit can be ground and used as spice.

This plant is quite easy to start from seed. Unfortunately, seeds are only viable for a narrow window of time after harvesting and are difficult to find. Also, don't confuse true star anise with Florida star anise (*Illicium floridanum*) or Japanese star anise (*Illicium anisatum*). *Those plants are similar in aroma and appearance and are easier to find. But they are potentially toxic and are* **not** considered safe to use as spice.

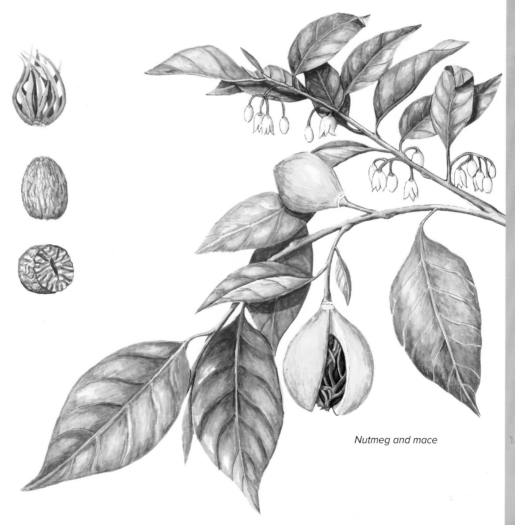

Nutmeg and mace

CONCLUSION
TENDING OUR GARDEN

As I write these closing words, it's spring. My poppies are up. The first cilantro is maturing. Mustard stands hip high, horseradish leaves are peaking out, and the saffron leaf tips are yellowing. I just planted fenugreek in my garden. Cumin, ginger, sesame, paprika, and others have been started in the greenhouse.

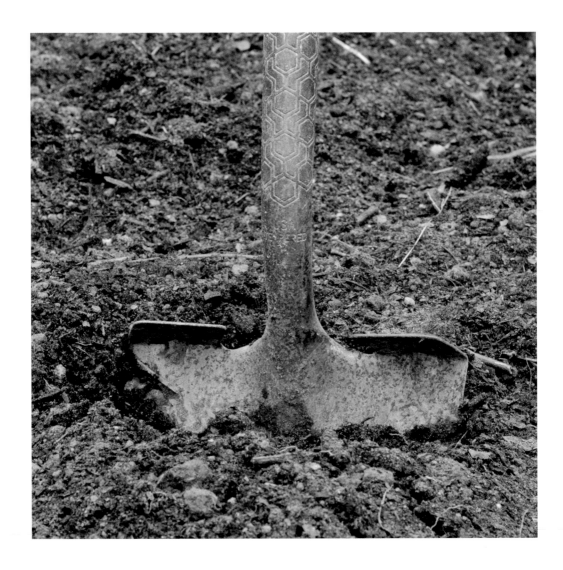

Also, the world is on lockdown to slow the spread of COVID-19. Hopefully, by the time you read this, the virus will be managed, though I know the ripple effects and the pain of personal losses will endure.

Through the pages of this book, I've done my best to share information about growing spices along with general gardening skills and tips. I've also tried to convey my gratitude for the cultures that made this astonishing variety of plants and their flavors, aromas, and health benefits possible.

There is no way I could cram everything I wanted to into the pages of this book nor is it necessary. The truth is, I'm just here to help you get started. These shared thoughts are seeds, to be planted or not. But while I have your attention, let me leave you with these final thoughts.

As COVID-19 has reminded us, we are more connected than we recognize in our daily lives. Nature has woven us together in ways that transcend our lack of proximity and cultural differences. That idea is frightening in terms of a virus, but to me it's also hopeful. It means we are never alone. Isolation is an illusion.

Growing a plant is easy. Growing an appreciation for the complex, intricate, and complicated natural and cultural diversity that made it possible in the first place takes more effort. Growing a kinder, more environmentally focused, and equitably distributed world—in which plants, insects, animals, and humans thrive—can seem an impossible task.

Yet I'm reminded of the age-old adage: Many hands make light work. Tending to our planet is no different than tending a garden. It takes knowledge paired with experience, tools, time, and earnest effort. Planet tending, though, is something we must all do together.

As one final meditation, know that within each seed, underground plant part, flower bud, or bit of bark, you hold our amazingly rich global cultural and natural history, an immensely interconnected present, and our shared future in your hands.

RESOURCES

Baker Creek Heirloom Seed Co.
2278 Baker Creek Road
Mansfield, MO 65704
Phone: (417) 924-8917
www.rareseeds.com

Companion Plants
7247 N. Coolville Ridge Road
Athens, OH 45701
Phone: (740) 592-4643
www.companionplants.com

Fast Growing Trees
2621 Old Nation Road
Fort Mill, SC 29715
www.fast-growing-trees.com

Hawaii Clean Seed
http://hawaiianorganicginger.com

Johnny's Selected Seeds
P.O. Box 299,
Waterville, ME 04903
Phone: (1-877) 564-6697
www.johnnyseeds.com

Logee's
141 North Street
Danielson, CT 06239
(860) 774-8038
www.logees.com

Raintree
408 Butts Road
Morton WA 98356
Phone: (1-800) 391-8892
www.raintreenursery.com

Seeds from Italy
P.O. Box 3908
Lawrence, KS 66046
Phone: (785) 748-0959
www.growitalian.com

Strictly Medicinal
P.O. Box 299
Williams, OR 97544
www.strictlymedicinalseeds.com

Territorial Seeds
20 Palmer Avenue,
Cottage Grove, OR 97424
Phone: (541) 942-0510
www.territorialseed.com

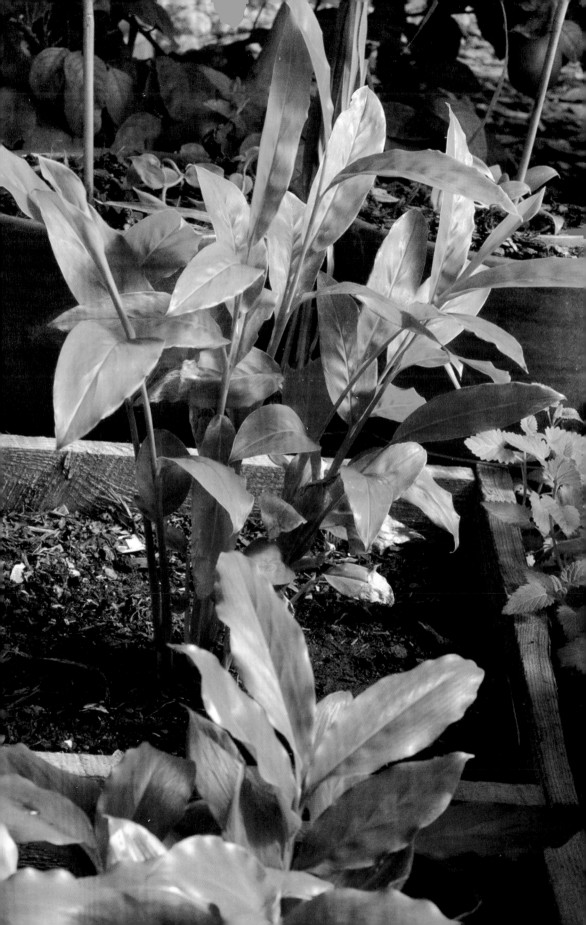

REFERENCES

BIBLIOGRAPHY

Caldicott, Chris and Carolyn Calidicott. The Spice Routes Recipes and Lore. California: SOMA Books, 2001.

Harding, Jennie. Herbs a Color Guide to Herbs and Herbal Healing. New York: Chartwell Books, 2017.

Heywood, V.H, editor. Flowering Plants of the World. New Jersey, Prentice Hall, 1985.

Ortiz, Elisabeth Lambert. The Encyclopedia of Herbs, Spices & Flavorings. New York: Dorling Kindersley, 1992.

Peter, K.V. Handbook of Herbs and Spices. Pennsylvania: Woodhead Publishing, 2012.

Rosengarten, Frederic. The Book of Spices. Pennsylvania: Livingston, 1969.

Sercarz, Lior Lev. Spice Companion. New York: Clarkson Potter, 2016.

Van Wyk, Ben-Erik. Culinary Herbs & Spices of the World. Chicago and London: The University of Chicago Press and Kew Publishing, 2013.

Zohary, Daniel, and Maria Hopf. Domestication of Plants in the Old World. Oxford: Oxford University Press, 2000

MAIN TEXT REFERENCES

i Prasad, Sahdea and Bharat B. Aggarwal "Chapter 13: Turmeric, the Golden Spice" from Herbal Medicine: Biomolecular and Clinical Aspects, 2nd edition ed. by Benzie IFF and Wachtel-Galor S. Boca Raton, FL: CRC Press/ Taylor & Francis; 2011.

MEDICINAL TIP REFERENCES

1 Panin, F., Serra, G., Pippia, P., & Moretti, M. D. L. (2002). Anti-inflammatory activity of linalool and linalyl acetate constituents of essential oils, 721–726.

2 Abascal, K., & Ahg, R. H. (2017). Cilantro— Culinary Herb or Miracle Medicinal Plant? (October 2012). https://doi.org/10.1089/ act.2012.185073.

3 Rahimi, R., Reza, M., & Ardekani, S. (2013). Medicinal Properties of Foeniculum Vulgare Mill in Traditional Iranian Medicine and Modern Phytotherapy, 19(1), 73–79. https://doi.org/ 10.1007/s11655-013-1327-0

4 Article, R. (2017). A Review of Its Physiology and Galactogogue Plants, 12(7). https://doi.org/ 10.1089/bfm.2017.0038

5 Grieve, M. (Maud). (1931). A modern herbal; the medicinal, culinary, cosmetic and economic properties, cultivation and folk-lore of herbs, grasses, fungi, shrubs, & trees with all their modern scientific uses. New York: Harcourt, Brace & company

6 Geberemeskel, G. A., Debebe, Y. G., & Nguse, N. A. (2019). Clinical Study Antidiabetic Effect of Fenugreek Seed Powder Solution (Trigonella foenum-graecum L.) on Hyperlipidemia in Diabetic Patients, 2019. https://doi.org/10.1155/ 2019/8507453

7 Majumdar, J., Chakraborty, P., Mitra, A., Sarkar, S., Bengal, W., Bengal, W., ... Diabetes, E. (n.d.). Fenugreek , A Potent Hypoglycaemic Herb Can Cause Central Hypothyroidism Via Leptin—A Threat To Diabetes Phytotherapy.

8 Grieve, M. (Maud). (1931). A modern herbal; the medicinal, culinary, cosmetic and economic properties, cultivation and folk-lore of herbs, grasses, fungi, shrubs, & trees with all their modern scientific uses. New York: Harcourt, Brace & Company

9 Yabanoglu, H., Akbulut, S., & Karakayali, F. (2012). Case Report Phytocontact Dermatitis due to Mustard Seed Mimicking Burn Injury: Report of a Case, 2012, 3–6. https://doi.org/10.1155/2012/5192151

10 Trial, D. P. C. (2015). Effect of the cumin cyminum L. Intake on Weight Loss, Metabolic Profiles and Biomarkers of Oxidative Stress in Overweight Subjects: A Randomized, (Cvd), 117–124. https://doi.org/10.1159/000373896

11 Al, I. A., Alhaider, A. A., Mossa, J. S., Al-s ohaibani, M. O., Al-yahya, M. A., Rafatullah, S., & Shaik, S. A. (2008). Gastroprotective Effect of an Aqueous Suspension of Black Cumin *Nigella sativa* on Necrotizing Agents-Induced Gastric Injury in Experimental Animals, 14(3), 128–134.

12 Wan, Y., Li, H., Fu, G., & Chen, X. (2015). The relationship of antioxidant components and antioxidant activity of sesame seed oil, (January). https://doi.org/10.1002/jsfa.7035

13 Khosravi-Boroujeni, Hossein. Can sesame consumption improve blood pressure? A systematic review and meta- analysis of controlled trials https://doi.org/10.1002/j

14 Derry, S., Asc, R., Cole, P., Tan, T., Ra, M., Derry, S., ... Ra, M. (2017). Topical capsaicin (high concentration) for chronic neuropathic pain in adults (Review), (1). https://doi.org/10.1002/14651858.CD007393.pub4.www.cochranelibrary.com

15 Khazdair, M. R., Boskabady, M. H., & Hosseini, M. (2015). The effects of *Crocus sativus* (saffron) and its constituents on nervous system: A review, 5(5), 376–391.

16 Ahmed, W., & Rashid, S. (2017). Functional and therapeutic potential of inulin: A comprehensive review. Critical Reviews in Food Science and Nutrition, 0(0), 1–13. https://doi.org/10.1080/10408398.2017.1355775

17 Herosimczyk, A., & O, M. (2007). Dietary chicory root and chicory inulin trigger changes in energetic metabolism , stress prevention and cytoskeletal proteins in the liver of growing pigs—a proteomic study, 1–12. https://doi.org/10.1111/jpn.12595

18 Zhu, Y., Anand, R., Geng, X., & Ding, Y. (2018). A mini review: garlic extract and vascular diseases. Neurological Research, 40(6), 421–425. https://doi.org/10.1080/01616412.2018.1451269

19 Ried, K. (2016). Garlic Lowers Blood Pressure in Hypertensive Individuals, Regulates Serum Cholesterol, and Stimulates Immunity: An Updated Meta-analysis and Review. The Journal of Nutrition, 146(2), 389S-396S. https://doi.org/10.3945/jn.114.202192

20 Chrubasik, S., Pittler, M. H., & Roufogalis, B. D. (2005). Zingiberis rhizoma: A comprehensive review on the ginger effect and efficacy profiles. Phytomedicine, 12(9), 684–701. https://doi.org/10.1016/j.phymed.2004.07.009

21 E., Smith, B. T., Gillespie, M., Eckl, V., Knepper, J., & Morton, C. (2019). 2018 ABC Herbal Sales MARKET REPORT, 62–73. Retrieved from www.herbalgram.org

22 Daily, J. W., Yang, M., & Park, S. (2016). Efficacy of Turmeric Extracts and Curcumin for Alleviating the Symptoms of Joint Arthritis: A Systematic Review and Meta-Analysis of Randomized Clinical Trials. Journal of Medicinal Food, 19(8), 717–729. https://doi.org/10.1089/jmf.2016.3705

23 Abrahams, S., Haylett, W. L., Johnson, G., Carr, J. A., & Bardien, S. (2019). Antioxidant effects of curcumin in models of neurodegeneration, aging, oxidative and nitrosative stress: A review. Neuroscience, 406, 1–21. https://doi.org/10.1016/j.neuroscience.2019.02.020

24 Ashokkumar, K., Murugan, M., Dhanya, M. K., & Warkentin, T. D. (2020). Botany, traditional uses, phytochemistry and biological activities of cardamom [*Elettaria cardamomum* (L.) Maton]—A critical review. Journal of Ethnopharmacology, 246, 112244. https://doi.org/10.1016/j.jep.2019.112244

25 Products, H. M., & Supplements, F. (2011). Herbal Monographs including Herbal Medicinal Products and Food Supplements. Department of Pharmacy University of Malta, p. 29

26 Shin, S. W. o., Ghimeray, A. K. uma., & Park, C. H. o. (2014). Investigation of total phenolic, total flavonoid, antioxidant and allyl isothiocyanate content in the different organs of Wasabi japonica grown in an organic system. African Journal of Traditional, Complementary, and Alternative Medicines: AJTCAM / African Networks on Ethnomedicines, 11(3), 38–45. https://doi.org/10.4314/ajtcam.v11i3.7

27 Subedi, L., Venkatesan, R., & Kim, S. Y. (2017). Neuroprotective and anti-inflammatory activities of allyl isothiocyanate through attenuation of JNK/NF-κB/TNF-α signaling. International Journal of Molecular Sciences, 18(7), 1–16. https://doi.org/10.3390/ijms18071423

28 Tlili, N., Elfalleh, W., Saadaoui, E., Khaldi, A., Triki, S., & Nasri, N. (2011). The caper (*Capparis* L.): Ethnopharmacology, phytochemical and pharmacological properties. Fitoterapia, 82(2), 93–101. https://doi.org/10.1016/j.fitote.2010.09.006

29 Nabavi, S. F., Maggi, F., Daglia, M., Habtemariam, S., Rastrelli, L., & Nabavi, S. M. (2016). Pharmacological Effects of *Capparis spinosa* L. Phytotherapy Research, 30(11), 1733–1744. https://doi.org/10.1002/ptr.5684

30 Khalil, E. A., Afifi, F. U., & Al-Hussaini, M. (2007). Evaluation of the wound healing effect of some Jordanian traditional medicinal plants formulated in Pluronic F127 using mice (Mus musculus). Journal of Ethnopharmacology, 109(1), 104–112. https://doi.org/10.1016/j.jep.2006.07.010

31 Klančnik, A., Zorko, Š., Toplak, N., Kovač, M., Bucar, F., Jeršek, B., & Smole Možina, S. (2018). Antiadhesion activity of juniper (*Juniperus communis* L.) preparations against *Campylobacter jejuni* evaluated with PCR-based methods. Phytotherapy Research, 32(3), 542–550. https://doi.org/10.1002/ptr.6005

32 Zhang, L., & L. Lokeshwar, B. (2012). Medicinal Properties of the Jamaican Pepper Plant *Pimenta dioica* and Allspice. Current Drug Targets, 13(14), 1900–1906. https://doi.org/10.2174/138945012804545641

33 Allen, R. W., Schwartzman, E., Baker, W. L., Coleman, C. I., & Phung, O. J. (2013). Cinnamon use in type 2 diabetes: An updated systematic review and meta-analysis. Annals of Family Medicine, 11(5), 452–459. https://doi.org/10.1370/afm.1517

34 Ogawa, K., Tashima, A., Sadakata, M., & Morinaga, O. (2018). Appetite-enhancing effects of vanilla flavours such as vanillin. Journal of Natural Medicines, 72(3), 798–802. https://doi.org/10.1007/s11418-018-1206-x

35 Takooree, H., Aumeeruddy, M. Z., Rengasamy, K. R. R., Venugopala, K. N., Jeewon, R., Zengin, G., & Mahomoodally, M. F. (2019). A systematic review on black pepper (*Piper nigrum* L.): from folk uses to pharmacological applications. Critical Reviews in Food Science and Nutrition, 59(0), S210–S243. https://doi.org/10.1080/10408398.2019.1565489

36 Meghwal, M., & Goswami, T. K. (2013). Piper nigrum and piperine: An update. Phytotherapy Research, 27(8), 1121–1130. https://doi.org/10.1002/ptr.4972

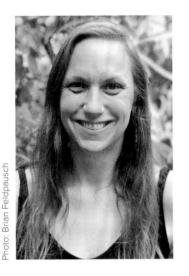

ABOUT THE AUTHOR
TASHA GREER

Tasha Greer is an "epicurean homesteader" and writer focused on simple, sustainable living. She gardens on about two acres and grows a large variety of annual and perennial edible, medicinal, and ecosystem support plants. She also keeps ducks, dairy goats, chickens, a pet turkey, worms, and (occasionally) pigs. She volunteers with gardening organizations in her community and teaches classes related to edible landscaping and organic gardening. When not growing food, cooking, or composting, Tasha's likely sitting on the garden swing with her partner, Matt Miles, surrounded by their two dogs and four cats. You can also find her at Simplestead.com.

ABOUT THE HERBALIST
LINDSEY FELDPAUSCH

Lindsey Feldpausch RH (AHG), is a clinical herbalist helping connect plants with the humans who need them. She believes in our innate ability to utilize the healing powers of plants, and one of her life's intentions is to kindle this belief in others. An experienced educator, she aims to balance both science and the magic of the natural world within in her teachings. Find out more at PlantMatters.org.

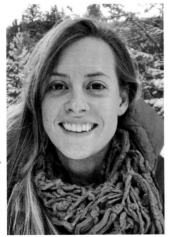

ABOUT THE ILLUSTRATOR
GRETA MOORE

This book was illustrated by Greta Moore, an illustrator and landscape designer in Bozeman, Montana. With a M.S in Ecological Landscape Design, she blends her passion for ecology with art to address climate change, improve food systems, restore habitats, create beautiful spaces, and bring plants and animals to life through watercolor paintings. She is also an avid backyard gardener and enjoys adventuring in the mountains and rivers of Montana. To see her work, visit gretacmoore.com.

ACKNOWLEDGMENTS

Listing an author's name on a book, along with the title, is like using Latin plant names for clarity. It allows libraries, booksellers, and readers to distinguish similarly titled books by author. However, I'm just one member of the team that created this book. Jessica Walliser was the book's driving force and facilitator. Lindsey, David, Nyle, Greta, Regina, Steve, Billie, John, and I each played parts creating, organizing, perfecting, and promoting it. We also each collaborated with others along the way. Collectively, we created something I am extremely proud to put my name on.

Thanks to Cody Britton and North Carolina Zoo (NCZoo.org) for research assistance and Tim Miles for photography advice. Also my deep appreciation goes to Matt Miles for making our everyday life an unbelievable luxury; Joy Millam for my first byline and years of encouragement; and my parents (Betty and Mike), my other "parents" (Steve, Tonya, Todd, Dave, Polly, Sue, and Tim), my extended family (Greer, Stevens, Whitaker, Miles, and Guevara clans), Surry County EMGVs, and the Round Peak beer/wine club for their long-time support. Finally, thank you for reading!

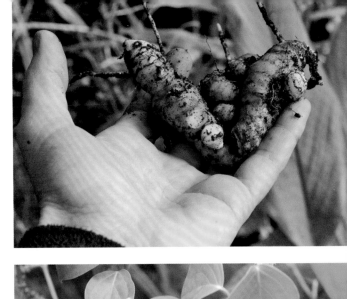
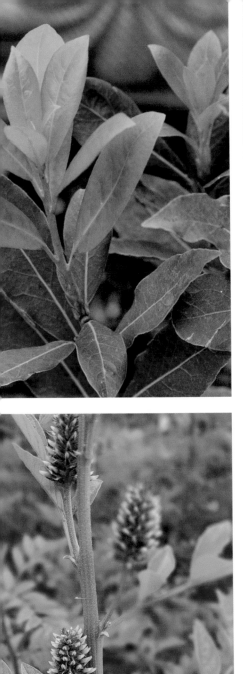
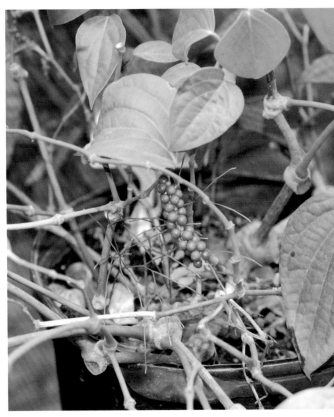
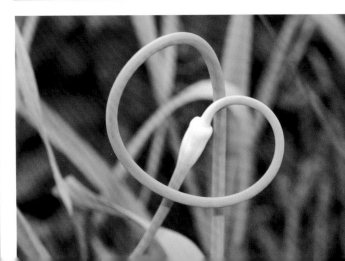

INDEX